T0185933

The Retina

Melvin J. Gouder

The Retina

A Guide to Self-Assessment

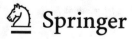 Springer

Melvin J. Gouder
Department of Ophthalmology
Mater Dei Hospital
Msida, Malta

ISBN 978-3-030-48593-1   ISBN 978-3-030-48591-7   (eBook)
https://doi.org/10.1007/978-3-030-48591-7

This Springer imprint is published by the registered company Springer Nature Switzerland AG
The registered company address is: Gewerbestrasse 11, 6330 Cham, Switzerland

Dedicated to Floyd Dylan Gouder, my son.

Preface

This book is aimed to assist and help the examinee. The idea behind this book was born decades ago when I was in my trainee years and always looking for books to help me succeed in my post-graduate exams in ophthalmic surgery. Then, the internet was in its infancy and learning was mainly through reading and revising and finding a source for self-testing in preparation for the exam. Those kinds of books were scanty. Though exam styles evolved and changed throughout the years, I still believed that multiple choice questions were a reliable source of testing one's knowledge. What I noticed then is that such books mostly offered a quick answer with no or minimal explanation related to the questions.

The idea behind this book is not to serve as a reference but to complement the equation and answer with detail about the subject matter being tested. This book provides 100+ questions on the retina mostly medical retina, but coming from the vitreoretinal field, I made sure to include a thorough chapter on the surgical aspect. Each question and answer should serve as an inspiration to stimulate the reader to seek further detail if it needs to be—perhaps in a reference text. MCQs help in problem solving and provide some form of reassurance in the pre-exam time hence increasing the chance of success. The final chapter is adorned with clinical photos of common and less common retinal disease one might expect to meet during an ophthalmological career.

Though RCOphth exams are still popular we have seen the emergence of the FEBO exam and many countries now provide their own post-graduate ophthalmic exams. This book is ideal for all these kinds of exams. Questions vary from simple straightforward ones to more complex subjects. Mixing the traditional with the modern is always more exciting and one can find this featured prominently throughout the whole book.

MCQs are always challenging and one has to accept that some may be controversial and ambiguous and a degree of misinterpretation is always expected.

Conceiving this book was not easy and hence I am indebted to certain people and colleagues who made all this possible. I am limitlessly indebted to Ms. Karen Grech, a talented book and paper conservator/restorer by profession whose ideas, though coming outside the medical field, have always been helpful and reassuring. Karen was crucial in helping me finish the book.

I am also indebted to Andrei Camenzuli, clinic manager and technical nurse at Saint James Eye Clinic in Malta, a private institution always at the forefront in providing the best medical and surgical ophthalmic care in Malta. And lastly but not least, I am indebted to my dad Joseph Gouder and my mum Angele Gouder who always believed in me and will do so *ad infinitum*.

Msida, Malta   Melvin J. Gouder

Contents

Abbreviations

AD	Autosomal dominant
AION	Anterior ischaemic optic neuropathy
AMN	Acute macular neuroretinopathy
AMPPE	Acute multifocal posterior pigment epitheliopathy
AR	Autosomal recessive
AV	Arteriovenous
BCVA	Best corrected visual acuity
BM	Bruch's membrane
CAR	Cancer-associated retinopathy
CC	Choriocapillaris
CHRPE	Congenital hypertrophy of the RPE
CNV	Choroidal neovascular membrane
CRAO	Central retinal artery obstruction
CRVO	Central retinal vein obstruction
CSR	Central serous retinopathy
DMO	Diabetic macular oedema
DR	Diabetic retinopathy
ELM	External limiting membrane
EOG	Electrooculogram
EOM	Extraocular muscle
FAF	Fundus autofluorescence
FAP	Familial adenomatous polyposis
FAZ	Foveal avascular zone
FEVR	Familial exudative vitreoretinopathy
FTMH	Full-thickness macular hole
GAG	Glycosaminoglycans
GCL	Ganglion cell layer
GRT	Giant retinal tear
HCQ	Hydroxychloroquin
i.v.	Intravenous
ICG	Indocyanine green

ILM	Inner limiting membrane
IOP	Intraocular pressure
IPL	Inner plexiform layer
IVFA	Intravenous fluorescein angiography
MEWDS	Multiple evanescent white dot syndrome
NAION	Non-Arteritic anterior ischaemic optic neuropathy
NFL	Nerve fibre layer
NVD	Neovascularisation at the disc
NVE	Neovascularisation elsewhere
NVI	Neovascularisation at the iris
OA	Ophthalmic artery
OCTA	Optical coherence tomography angiogram
ONL	Outer nuclear layer
OPL	Outer plexiform layer
PAMM	Paracentral acute middle maculopathy
PCV	Polypoidal choroidal vasculopathy
PDR	Proliferative diabetic retinopathy
PED	Posterior epithelial detachment
PHM	Posterior hyaloid membrane
PR	Photoreceptors
prn	Pro re nata
PXE	Pseudoxanthoma elasticum
RAPD	Relative afferent pupillary defect
ROP	Retinopathy of prematurity
RP	Retinitis pigmentosa
RPE	Retinal pigment epithelium
SLO	Scanning laser ophthalmoscopy
SPCA	Short posterior ciliary artery
VEGF	Vascular endothelial growth factor
VHL	Von Hippel–Lindau disease
WWOP	White without pressure
WWP	White with pressure
XLJR	X-linked juvenile retinoschisis

Chapter 1
Basic Anatomy, Embryology and Physiology of the Retina

1. Retinal histology:

   (a) its thickness does not vary
   (b) the innermost layer is the retinal ganglion cell layer
   (c) the outermost layer is also the outermost layer of the neuroretina
   (d) bruch's membrane is associated with the RPE
   (e) the Umbo is in the centre of the fovea.

2. Retina and vitreous embryology [1]:

   (a) The retina is derived from the optic vesicle
   (b) It is an out-pouching of the embryonic midbrain
   (c) The vitreous is mainly composed of GAG and collagen
   (d) Vitreous and choroid are derived from mesenchyme
   (e) Mittendorf dot and Bergmeister papilla are remnants of the hyaloid artery.

3. Retina and vitreous embryology:

   (a) Retina forms from neuroectoderm
   (b) the hyaloid artery is derived from the vascular mesoderm
   (c) sensory retina forms from the inner layer of the optic cup
   (d) RPE is formed from the outer layer of optic cup
   (e) the hyaloid artery is derived from the ophthalmic artery.

4. The vitreous [2]:

   (a) Is composed of two main areas: the vitreous core and cortical vitreous.
   (b) Forms 80% of the eye volume
   (c) The anterior retrolental vitreous is condensed

© Springer Nature Switzerland AG 2020
M. J. Gouder, *The Retina*, https://doi.org/10.1007/978-3-030-48591-7_1

(d) The vitreous base is closely associated with the zonular fibres of the lens
(e) It is high in ascorbate levels.

5. The ora serrata:

(a) It is the border between the peripheral retina and pars plana
(b) It is a very smooth transition of the periphery of the retina
(c) Retinal tears are associated with meridional folds
(d) Dentate processes are teeth-like extensions of retina onto the pars plana
(e) Tears in the ora serrata area may be associated with pigmentary changes.

6. The fovea [3]:

(a) The fovea has no rods
(b) The central fovea is called the foveola
(c) In the fovea the inner cellular layers of the retina are displaced laterally
(d) RPE is densest at this region
(e) Cones in the fovea are predominately yellow- and blue-sensitive.

7. RPE histology [4];

(a) It is sometimes multilayered
(b) Melanosomes are spread evenly in the cell
(c) The cell base is firmly associated with the choroidal vasculature
(d) Their apices are in contact with the outer segments of the photoreceptors
(e) Melanosomes are abundant in the cells lying beneath the fovea.

8. RPE physiology [6, 7];

(a) RPE forms the outer blood-retinal layer
(b) RPE, being a monolayer, rarely heals by scarring
(c) Integral in recycling visual pigment
(d) Phagocytosis is continuous
(e) Is able to regenerate.

9. Bruch's membrane;

(a) Is pentalaminar
(b) Prone to calcify in pathologic processes
(c) Essential in keeping the retina healthy
(d) Suppresses the formation of choroidal neovascular membranes
(e) Is fractured in Angioid streaks.

10. Choroid;

    (a) Is supplied mainly by the anterior ciliary arteries
    (b) The choriocapillaris circulation is high pressure
    (c) Gets thinner away from the macular area
    (d) Is highly pigmented
    (e) Thickness changes are associated with ocular disease.

11. Choroidal anatomy [5];

    (a) Choroid is tightly adhered to the sclera
    (b) Up to ten vortex veins provide choroidal drainage
    (c) Innervated by the long and short ciliary nerves
    (d) Haller's and Sattler's layer are vascular
    (e) There is a low pressure blood flow in the choriocapillaris.

12. Choroidal physiology;

    (a) Choroidal vasculature supplies the outer retina
    (b) The photoreceptors of the retina are highly active
    (c) The choroid has a high blood flow
    (d) Venous blood exiting the choroid has a low oxygen tension
    (e) The choroid is a heat sink.

13. Sclera;

    (a) Uniform thickness throughout
    (b) Is permeable to drugs injected around the eye
    (c) Derived from neural crest
    (d) Composed of collagen, elastic fibres and proteoglycans
    (e) Pigmentation is common.

1   Answers

  1. FFFTT
  2. TFFTT
  3. TTTTT
  4. TTTFT
  5. TFFTT
  6. FTTTF
  7. FFFTT
  8. TFTTF

9. TTTTT
10. FFTTT
11. FFTTT
12. TTTFT
13. FTTTT.

2   Answers in Detail

1. FFFTT

Retinal thickness varies throughout but it shows greatest variation centrally i.e. around the macula. It is thinnest at the foveal floor (<60 microns) than gets thicker immediately around the macula (~330 microns). Away from the macula it rapidly thins until the equator (~150 microns) and at the ora serrata it is ~160 microns.

Retinal layers from inside out—ILM-RNFL-GCL-IPL-INL-OPL-ONL-ELM-PR-RPE hence the RPE is the outermost layer and the ILM is the innermost layer. The RPE is attached to BM. The Umbo is the central part of the fovea.

2. TFFTT

The retina is derived from the optic vesicle which is an out-pouching of the embryonic forebrain. The mature vitreous is mainly composed of water (99%). The rest is made up of hyaluronic acid collagen type 2, hyalocytes, inorganic salts and ascorbic acid and has a pH of 7.5. The vitreous and choroid are derived from mesenchyme, the retina from the neuroectoderm and the cornea from surface ectoderm (corneal epithelium) and mesenchyme (corneal stroma). Mittendorf dot is a small opacity on the posterior aspect of the lens whereas a Bergmeister papilla is a tuft of fibrous tissue on the optic nerve head—all remnants of the hyaloid artery.

3. TTTTT

The retina forms from neuroectoderm. The hyaloid artery is derived from the vascular mesoderm.

Sensory retina forms from the inner layer of the optic cup whereas the RPE is formed from the outer layer of the optic cup.

The hyaloid artery is derived from the ophthalmic artery which in adults is a branch of the internal carotid artery. When the hyaloid artery regresses it leaves a clear central zone in the vitreous called Cloquet's canal. If the artery does not regress it can remain in the vitreous as a persistent hyaloid artery.

4. TTTFT

The vitreous is made up of the central (or core) and the peripheral (cortical) vitreous. It forms 80 percent of the eye volume and made up of hydrated hyaluronic acid with suspended collagen fibrils. The anterior vitreous behind the lens is made up of condensed collagen fibres that are attached to the posterior capsule of the lens—ligament of Weiger. Berger space is the potential space bordering this ligament. The vitreous is particularly attached firmly at the vitreous base, lens capsule, retinal vessels, optic nerve and macula. Ascorbic acid, which is very high in the lens, has a protective role in the lens. Vitrectomy—which removes most of the vitreous from the eye—increases the chance of lenticular opacities in the post-op period (typically nuclear sclerosis).

5. TFFTT

The peripheral retina extends anteriorly and ends in the ora serrata. It is an irregular, 'serrated' area of transition with specific anatomic features. Meridional folds are areas of excess retina bulging slightly into the vitreous where at its base can be weak and retinal tears occur. A dentate process (dentate means tooth) is an area of real parts of the retina jutting into the pars plana like a spear. At the ora serrata region the pigmented epithelium of the retina transitions into the outer pigmented epithelium of the ciliary body and the inner portion of the retina transitions into the non-pigmented epithelium of the ciliary body.

Retinal RPE → outer pigment epithelium of the ciliary body and iris
Neurosensory Retina. → inner non-pigmented epithelium of the ciliary body.

6. FTTTF

Actually it is the foveola, or the central fovea that is devoid of rods. Rods reach maximal density around 4 mm from the foveal centre. The fovea is rich in red- and green-sensitive cones and cones density decrease away from the fovea explaining the decrease in the visual acuity away from fixation. In the fovea the inner cellular layers of the retina are displaced laterally so as light scatter is reduced. Beneath the fovea, RPE density is very high as this is a very active metabolic region.

   The foveola is the thinnest part of the retina. Apart from cones there are also Muller cells and their processes.

7. FFFTT

The RPE cell is a hexagonal cell which is very metabolically active. It is derived from the outer layer of the optic cup. The RPE cell layer is a monolayer and beneath the fovea it is not only the density that changes (increases) but also the shape, becoming taller and thinner so more of them fit per unit area. Melanosomes are denser towards the cell's apex next to the photoreceptors. The nucleus of the cell is more commonly found at the outer area next to the Bruch's membrane.

8. TFTTF

Functions and features of the RPE:

I.   Forms the outer blood-retina layer (tight junctions between cells are called zonulae occludens—most densely situated near the apex).
II.   Development of photoreceptors during embryogenesis.

III. This outer blood-retina layer prevents extracellular fluid leaking into the sub-retinal space from the choriocapillaris found beneath the Bruch membrane.

IV.   Actively pumps water and ions out of the sub-retinal space (provided there are no tears in the neurosensory retina a lot of sub-retinal fluid can be resorbed in a couple of hours. In normal situations the RPE keeps the sub-retinal space free from water.

V.   The RPE is intimately attached to the Bruch's membrane beneath by the help of osmotic and hydrostatic pressure and hemidesmosomes.

VI.   Continuous phagocytosis and re-cycling of the outer photoreceptor layer. Intra-RPE lysosomes degrade the engulfed outer PR disc fragments hence maintaining turn over of PR. The rods shed discs at night and the cones shed them at dusk.

VII. Promotes a health retina by taking care of waste products and allowing transport of healthy metabolites towards the neuroretina.

VIII. Uptake, transport, storage, metabolism and isomerization of vitamin A.

IX.   Absorption of stray light by melanin to control light scatter.

9. TTTTT

Basically, the Bruch's membrane, as seen through the electron microscope is made up of 5 layers. It is enveloped between the RPE and the choroid choriocapillaris. Histopathological changes to the basic Bruch's membrane leads to the pathogenesis of many diseases. For example calcification of the Bruch's membrane can lead to fractures and CNV formation such as what happens in angioid streaks.

Bruch's Membrane Layers	Thickness (microns)
RPE basal lamina	0.3
Inner collagenous layer	1.5
Band of elastic fibres	0.8
Outer collagenous layer	0.7
Choriocapillaris basal lamina	0.1

10. FFTTT

The choroid, is the vascular layer of the eye, containing connective tissues, and is sandwiched between the retina and sclera. The choroid is thickest at the submacular area (at 0.2 mm), while near the ora serrata it narrows to 0.1 mm where it is the thinnest. The choroid provides oxygen and nourishment to the outer layers of the retina. Along with the ciliary body and iris, the choroid forms the uveal tract.

The choroid receives its blood supply primarily from the posterior ciliary branches of the ophthalmic artery but there is also some supply from the recurrent anterior ciliary arteries. Pachychoroid means thick choroid where leptochoroid means thin choroid and both can be signs of disease.

11. FFTTT

The choroid adheres only loosely to the sclera over most of its area, and as a consequence, the choroid is easily separated from the sclera by either haemorrhage or serous fluid. The only points at which the choroid is fixed are the optic nerve and at the vortex veins. Attachment of the choroid to the sclera at the vortex veins explains the classic quadrantic appearance of choroidal detachments. Four or five vortex veins provide the choroid's venous drainage. The nerve supply of the choroid is derived from the long and short ciliary nerves.

Trigeminal nerve (CN V1) —>Nasociliary nerves —>long ciliary nerves. (sensory + sympathetic)

Oculomotor nerve (CNIII) —>ciliary ganglion —>short ciliary nerves (sympathetic and parasympathetic fibres)

Haller's layer—the outer large caliber choroidal vessels
Sattler's layer—smaller diameter vessels and pre-capillary arterioles

There is a low pressure blood flow in the choriocapillaris.

Interspersed with the blood vessels are melanocytes, nevus cells, and nerves. These blood vessels possess an outer adventitial layer, an intermediate smooth muscle layer, and an internal elastic lamina. They are not fenestrated and as a result do not leak dye during fluorescein angiography.

Sattler's layer is deep to Haller's layer and is composed of medium-sized blood vessels, melanocytes, fibroblasts, lymphocytes, mast cells, and supporting collagen fibres. Within Sattler's layer, arteries gradually decrease in caliber and form arterioles. In the process, the arteries lose their muscularis layer and their internal elastic laminae. Like the vessels of Haller's layer, the vessels of Sattler's layer are not fenestrated and do not leak fluorescein.

The choriocapillaris is a layer of capillaries that is immediately adjacent to Bruch's membrane. The diameter of the capillaries is relatively large and measures between 25 and 50 μm. These capillaries are fenestrated and therefore are permeable to large molecules, including fluorescein. On fluorescein angiography, the diffuse fluorescence of the choroid is primarily due to the leakage of fluorescein from the choriocapillaris. The choriocapillaris extends from the edge of the optic disc to the ora serrata.

12. TTTFT

The choroidal vasculature supplies the retina and is responsible for supplying 90% of retinal oxygen needs—the photoreceptors being one of the most metabolically active cells of the retina. The oxygen tension in the venous outflow of the choroid still has a high oxygen tension hence prone to oxidative damage. Since blood flow is fast, the choroid tends to 'cool' the retina by acting as a heat sink in removing thermal energy accumulating by light absorption.

13. FTTTT

The sclera forms the posterior 5/6 of the eye with the remainder made up of the cornea. It is white and opaque but its colour is determined by pigmentation, deposits and circulation status. It is hydrophilic and permeable to certain drugs injected in the subtenon space as a form of local medication. Embryologically derived from neural crest and composed mainly of collagen, a few elastic fibres embedded in proteoglycans. Dark skinned individuals may have a darker sclera. Thin sclera in kids give it a greyish tone from the choroid.

References

1. Cassin B, Solomon S. Dictionary of eye terminology. Gainesville, Florida: Triad Publishing Company; 1990.
2. Romer AS, Parsons TS. The vertebrate body. Philadelphia, PA: Holt-Saunders International; 1977. p. 461. ISBN 978-0-03-910284-5.
3. Development of the eye by Victoria Ort, Ph.D and David Howard, M.D. http://education.med. nyu.edu/courses/macrostructure/lectures/lec_images/eye.html.
4. LifeMap Science, Inc. Embryonic and postnatal development of the eye. https://discovery.life-mapsc.com/in-vivo-development/eye.
5. Gilbert SF. Developmental Biology. 6th edition. Sunderland (MA): Sinauer Associates; 2000. Development of the Vertebrate Eye. Available from: https://www.ncbi.nlm.nih.gov/books/ NBK10024/.
6. Sensory reception: human vision: structure and function of the human eye, vol. 27. Encyclopaedia Britannica; 1987. p. 174.
7. Strauss O. The retinal pigment epithelium in visual function. Physiol Rev. 2005;85:845–81.

Chapter 2
Retinal Testing and Imaging

1. Direct Ophthalmoscopy [1];

    (a) is better than indirect ophthalmoscopy
    (b) is a monocular test
    (c) high-magnification up to ×15
    (d) small field of view
    (e) it is great for the periphery.

2. Indirect Ophthalmoscopy;

    (a) provides a low magnification and an inverted image
    (b) provides a stereoscopic image
    (c) optimum field of view
    (d) easy to master
    (e) is a non-contact test.

3. The three-mirror lens;

    (a) provides high-resolution images
    (b) gives high magnification view of the retina
    (c) non-inverted images
    (d) the apical smallest mirror is used for the equatorial retina
    (e) since the contact lens touches the cornea, total internal reflection issues are obliterated.

4. Fundus photos:

    (a) mydriasis is always needed
    (b) gives information only to central retina

© Springer Nature Switzerland AG 2020
M. J. Gouder, *The Retina*, https://doi.org/10.1007/978-3-030-48591-7_2

(c) cataracts do not hinder photo capture
(d) different filters can be used
(e) is a cheap test.

5. IVFA [3]:

(a) fluorescein enters the ocular circulation from the internal carotid artery via the ophthalmic artery
(b) venous stage at 1 min
(c) choroidal flush occurs before retinal filling
(d) involves the injection of 25 cm^3 of sodium fluorescein into a vein in the arm or hand.
(e) patient may feel nauseous once the dye is injected.

6. Physics of IVFA:

(a) the retina is illuminated by blue light
(b) the camera allows yellow-green light from the retina
(c) the filters used are called interference bandpass filters
(d) autofluorescence is fluorescence from the eye which occurs without injection of the dye
(e) pseudofluorescence means non-fluorescent light is imaged.

7. Causes of hyperfluorescence in IVFA:

(a) leakage of fluid
(b) staining of tissues
(c) blocking in ischaemia
(d) transmission, or window, defect
(e) autofluorescence.

8. Causes of hypofluorescence in IVFA [4]:

(a) ischaemia
(b) retinal embolism
(c) macroaneurysms
(d) optic disc drusen
(e) myopic chorioretinal degeneration.

9. Indocyanine green (ICG) [8, 9]:

(a) is fat-soluble
(b) almost completely protein-bound after injection
(c) leaks profusely through the choriocapillaris
(d) ICG is metabolised in the liver and excreted via bile.
(e) fluoresces very efficiently.

10. Indications for ICG angiography include the following:

   (a) CNV
   (b) pigment epithelial detachment (PED)
   (c) polypoidal choroidal vasculopathy (PCV)
   (d) central serous chorioretinopathy
   (e) choroidal inflammatory conditions.

11. Advantages of OCT Angiography over IVFA [2]:

   (a) no dye is used
   (b) cheaper test
   (c) can identify different layers of the retina
   (d) higher definition images
   (e) non-invasive.

12. B-Scan ultrasonography [5, 6]:

   (a) B stands for "brightness"
   (b) no need to use topical anaesthesia
   (c) useful in detecting retinal detachment in the presence of dense vitreous haemorrhage
   (d) increasing the gain setting increases the resolution
   (e) only useful in intraocular pathology.

13. The following are true about electroretinogram [7]:

   (a) the a-wave is produced by the photoreceptors
   (b) the b-wave is produced by the ganglion cells
   (c) c-wave is produced by the retinal pigment epithelium
   (d) different light frequencies can be used to separate rod and cone response
   (e) it is useful for detecting early Best's disease.

14. The electrooculogram (EOG):

   (a) measures the electrical potential between the front and the back of the eye
   (b) has a resting potential of 40 mV
   (c) is abnormal in optic nerve disease
   (d) is abnormal in Best's disease even before the onset of visual symptoms
   (e) can be measured using the Arden Index which is the ratio of dark trough to light rise.

15. The following statements are true:

   (a) ERG is diagnostic of Stargardt's disease
   (b) amplitude of ERG is reduced in carriers of choroideremia

(c) EOG light peak to dark trough ratio is normal in adult-onset foveomacular dystrophy

(d) ERG is diagnostic of Leber's congenital amaurosis

(e) ERG is useful in detecting carrier of X-linked retinitis pigmentosa.

16. The following are true in relation to full-field ERG [7]:

(a) in carotid artery occlusion (CRAO) there is a reduced b-wave greater than a-wave amplitudes

(b) in hypertension and arteriosclerosis there is initially reduced oscillatory potentials followed by reduced a- and b-wave amplitudes

(c) in thioridazine toxicity there is decreased photopic and scotopic a- and b-wave responses

(d) in hydroxychloroquine toxicity there is normal ERG responses unless presence of advanced retinopathy; cone function initially more affected than rod function

(e) in Cone dystrophy there is markedly depressed photopic response and less affected scotopic response.

1   Answers

1. FTTTF
2. TTTTF
3. TFTFT
4. FFFTF
5. TFTTT
6. TTTTT
7. TTFTT
8. TTTFF
9. FTFTF
10. TTTTT
11. TFTTT
12. TFTFF
13. TFTTF
14. TFFTF
15. FFTTT
16. TTTTT.

2 Answers in Detail

1. FTTTF

Direct ophthalmoscopy also sometimes known as fundoscopy provides a vertical, monocular high magnification image mostly used to examine the central retina, optic disc and nearby vessels (the eye grounds). However, it provides a very small field of view ranging from 5–8 degrees—similar to the image obtained using a telephoto lens in photography. So, this requires a lot of ocular steering to view peripheral areas but as such is not used to examine the retinal periphery. It is popular with medics and other non-ophthalmic specialists mainly to assess the eye from a systemic point of view (such as to rule out an optic disc swelling, obtain some macular information in diabetic macular oedema or even used as light source to elicit pupillary reflexes).

2. TTTTF

Indirect Ophthalmoscopy can be carried out with a head mounted instrument or incorporated during slit-lamp analysis using a 90D, 90D wide field, 78D or a 60D lens. The following table shows the main differences between direct and indirect ophthalmoscopy (Table 1).

In indirect ophthalmoscopy various condensing lenses can be used typically and commonly the 20D and 28D in the head mounted type instrument and the 90D (wide-field option available) and 78D, the latter more for macular assessment as it gives a more magnified view of the macula. A 20D lens gives a magnification of $-60/20D = -3$ (see Table 2) with the *minus* sign indicating it is an inverted image. Hence a 28D lens which is typically used in paediatric fundus examinations gives a better field of view but a smaller magnification. In slit-lamp indirect ophthalmoscopy there is the advantage that magnification can be changed from the slit-lamp itself.

3. TFTFF

The three-mirror lens (like the Goldmann three-mirror lens) is a form of contact direct ophthalmoscopy that is essential to examine in detail the central and

Table 1 Comparison between direct and indirect ophthalmoscopy

Direct ophthalmoscopy	Indirect ophthalmoscopy
High magnification ($\times 15$)	Low magnification ($\times 3$ with 20D condensing lens)
Low field of view	High field of view
Monocular	Binocular
2D image	3D image (stereoscopic image)
Erect image	Inverted image (and reversed)
Limited peripheral retina view	Full peripheral retina view up to ora errata (can be combined with scleral depressor for a better view)
No need to darken room	Better if room is darkened
Clinician has to be very near the patient	Clinician some distance away (arms length)

Table 2 Comparison of various condensing lenses

Lens	Magnification	Field of view (degrees)	Notes
20D	×3	45	Most commonly used
28D	×2.27	53	Used in paediatrics and through a small pupil
40D	×1.5	65	Used in uncooperative patients to obtain a quick fundus overview
Panretinal 2.2	×2.68	56	Combines magnification nearly that of the 20D lens with a field of view approaching that of the 30D lens.

Table 3 The Goldmann three-mirror lens

1. Central lens	Round	30 degree upright view
2. Equatorial mirror	Largest mirror	From 30 degrees to equator
3. Peripheral mirror	Intermediate sized	From equator to ora serrata
4. Gonioscopy mirror	Smallest and dome—shaped	Extreme retinal periphery, Pars plana, gonioscopy

peripheral retina. It provides high-resolution images with no magnification (image can be magnified by using slit-lamp magnification). A huge advantage is that it provides non inverted images and the central portion of the lens gives a field of view of up to 20 degrees. The other three mirrors can be used to evaluate the mid periphery and the peripheral retina with the apical smallest mirror ideal also for gonioscopic analysis (Table 3).

4. FFFTF

Fundus photography involves photographing the fundus. Specialised fundus cameras consisting of an intricate microscope attached to a flash enabled camera are used in fundus photography. The main structures that can be visualised on a fundus photo are the central and peripheral retina, optic disc and macula. Fundus photography can be performed with coloured filters, or with specialised dyes including fluorescein (IVFA) and indocyanine green (ICG angiography)

Advantages of using a fundus camera:

– quick and easy to use and master
– observes a larger retinal field at any one time compares to ophthalmoscopy
– modern cameras are non-mydriatic
– image can be saved and used for monitoring of disease and teaching
– spectrum of filters can be used to obtain more detail and contrast
– the use of dyes such as fluorescein and ICG can be used to get physiological information about the retina
– different magnification options to focus on a particular area

– composite images possible to access peripheral retina
– 3-D imaging possible with modern cameras.

Disadvantages of using a fundus camera:

- difficulty observing and assessing abnormalities such a cotton wool spots due to lack of depth appreciation on images
- less image clarity than indirect ophthalmoscopy
- cataracts, vitreous opacities can hinder photographic access of the fundus
- artefact error may produce unusual images
- lack of portability
- expensive machine.

5. TFTTT

Fluorescein enters the ocular circulation from the internal carotid artery via the ophthalmic artery. The ophthalmic artery (OA) is the first branch of the internal carotid artery distal to the cavernous sinus. The ophthalmic artery supplies the choroid via the short posterior ciliary arteries (SPCA) and the retina via the central retinal artery (CRA), however, the route to the choroid is typically less circuitous than the route to the retina. This accounts for the short delay between the "choroidal flush" and retinal filling.

Approximate normal circuitry filling time:

- 0 seconds—injection of fluorescein
- 9.5 seconds—posterior ciliary arteries
- 10 seconds—choroidal flush (or "pre-arterial phase")
- 10–12 seconds—retinal arterial stage
- 13 seconds—capillary transition stage
- 14–15 seconds—early venous stage (or "laminar stage", "arterial-venous stage")
- 16–17 seconds—venous stage
- 18–20 seconds—late venous stage
- 5 minutes—late staining.

Nausea is a common sensation as the dye reaches the midbrain. It is benign.

6. TTTTT

In IVFA:

Equipment-

- Exciter filter: Allows only blue light to illuminate the retina. Depending on the specific filter, the excitation wavelength hitting the retina will be between 465 and 490 nm. Most filters only allow light through at a wavelength of 490 nm.

- Barrier filter: Allows only yellow-green light (from the fluorescence) to reach the camera. Both filters are interference bandpass filters, which means they block out all light except that at a specific wavelength. The barrier filter only allows light with a wavelength of 525 nm, but depending on the filter it can be anywhere from 520–530 nm.
- Fundus camera, either digital or with camera body containing black and white, or slide positive film.

Technique-

- Baseline colour (colour fundus photo) and black and white red-free filtered images are taken prior to injection. The black and white images are filtered red-free (a green filter) to increase contrast and often gives a better image of the fundus than the colour image.
- A 6-second bolus injection of 2–5 cm^3 of sodium fluorescein into a vein in the arm or hand.
- A series of black-and-white or digital photographs are taken of the retina before and after the fluorescein reaches the retinal circulation (approximately 10 seconds after injection). The early images allow for the recognition of autofluorescence of the retinal tissues. Photos are taken approximately once every second for about 20 seconds, then less often. A delayed image is obtained at 5 and 10 minutes. Some doctors like to see a 15-minute image as well.
- A barrier filter is placed in the camera so only the fluorescent, yellow-green light (530 nm) is recorded. The camera may however pick up signals from pseudofluorescence or autofluorescence. In pseudofluorescence, non-fluorescent light is imaged. This occurs when blue light reflected from the retina passes through the filter. This is generally a problem with older filters, and annual replacement of these filters is recommended. In autofluorescence, fluorescence from the eye occurs without injection of the dye. This may be seen with optic nerve head drusen, astrocytic hamartoma, or calcific scarring.
- Black-and-white photos give better contrast than colour photos, which aren't necessary because the filter transmits only one colour of light.

7. TTFTT

Causes of hyperfluorescence in IVFA;

- leakage
- staining
- pooling
- transmission, or window defect
- autofluorescence.

Leakage refers to the gradual, marked increase in fluorescence throughout the angiogram when fluorescein molecules seep through the pigment epithelium into the subretinal space or neurosensory retina, out of retinal blood vessels into the retinal interstitium, or from retinal neovascularization into the vitreous. The borders of hyperfluorescence become increasingly blurred and fuzzy, and the greatest intensity of hyperfluorescence is found in the late phases of the study, when the only significant fluorescein dye remaining in the eye is extravascular. Leakage occurs, for example, in CNV, in microaneurysms, in telangiectatic capillaries, in diabetic macular oedema, and in neovascularization of the disc.

Staining refers to a pattern of hyperfluorescence where the fluorescence gradually increases in intensity through transit views and persists in late views, but its borders remain *fixed* throughout the angiogram. Staining results from fluorescein entry into a solid tissue or similar material that retains the fluorescein, such as a scar, drusen, optic nerve tissue, or sclera.

Pooling refers to the accumulation of fluorescein in a fluid-filled space in the retina or choroid. At the beginning of the angiogram, the fluid in this abnormal space contains no fluorescein and is not visible. As fluorescein leaks into the space, the margins of the space trap the fluorescein and appear distinct, as seen, for example, in an RPE detachment, in central serous chorioretinopathy (CSR). As more fluorescein enters the space, the entire area fluoresces.

A *transmission defect*, or *window defect*, refers to a view of the normal choroidal fluorescence through a defect in the pigment or loss of pigment in the RPE. In a transmission defect, the hyperfluorescence occurs early, corresponding to filling of the choroidal circulation, and reaches its greatest intensity with the peak of choroidal filling. The fluorescence does not increase in size or shape and usually fades in the late phases of the angiogram, as the choroidal fluorescence becomes diluted by blood that does not contain fluorescein. The fluorescein remains in the choroid and does not enter the retina.

Autofluorescence describes the appearance of fluorescence from the fundus captured *prior* to intravenous fluorescein injection. It is seen with structures that naturally fluoresce, such as optic nerve drusen and lipofuscin.

8. TTTFF

*Hypo*fluorescence occurs when normal fluorescence is reduced or absent; it is present in 2 major patterns:

- blocked fluorescence
- vascular filling defect.

Vascular filling defects occur where the retinal or choroidal vessels do not fill properly, as in non perfusion of an artery, vein, or capillary in the retina or choroid. These defects produce either a delay or a complete absence in filling of the involved vessels.

Blocked fluorescence occurs when the stimulation or visualisation of the fluorescein is blocked by fibrous tissue or another barrier, such as pigment or blood, producing an absence of normal retinal or choroidal fluorescence in the area.

Blocked fluorescence is most easily differentiated from hypofluorescence due to hypoperfusion by evaluating the ophthalmoscopic view, where a lesion is usually visible that corresponds to the area of blocked fluorescence. If no corresponding area is visible clinically, then it is likely an area of vascular filling defect and not blocked fluorescence. By evaluating the level of the blocked fluorescence in relation to the retinal circulation, one can determine how deep the lesion resides. For example, when lesions block the choroidal circulation but retinal vessels are present over this blocking defect, then the lesions are above the choroid and below the retinal vessels.

9. FTFTF

Indocyanine green (ICG) is a water-soluble, tricarbocyanine dye with a molecular weight of 775 daltons that is almost completely protein-bound (98%) after intravenous injection. Because it is protein-bound, diffusion through the small fenestrations of the choriocapillaris is limited. The retention of ICG in the choroidal circulation, coupled with low permeability, makes ICG angiography ideal for imaging choroidal circulation. ICG is metabolised in the liver and excreted into the bile.

ICG fluoresces in the near-infrared range (790–805 nm). Thus, it can be injected immediately before or after FA. Because its fluorescence efficacy is only 4% that of fluorescein dye, it can be detected only with specialised infrared video angiography using modified fundus cameras, a digital imaging system, or a scanning laser ophthalmoscope (SLO). ICG angiography uses a diode laser illumination system with an output of 805 nm and barrier filters at 500 and 810 nm.

10. TTTTT

Because of its longer operating wavelength, a theoretical advantage of ICG is its ability to fluoresce better through pigment, fluid, lipid, and haemorrhage than fluorescein dye, thereby increasing the possibility of detecting abnormalities such as CNV that may be blocked by an overlying thin, subretinal haemorrhage or hyperplastic RPE on a traditional fluorescein angiogram. This allows enhanced imaging in occult CNV and PED. CNV appears on ICG angiography as a plaque, a focal hot spot, or a combination of both. *Plaques* are usually formed by late-staining vessels and usually correspond to occult CNV. *Focal hot spots* are well-delineated fluorescent spots less than 1 disc diameter in size that typically indicate retinal angiomatous proliferations (RAP) and polypoidal vasculopathy, which are variants of CNV. However, ICG used in eyes with these features has not consistently produced images of well-defined CNV that look like traditional CNV on FA.

ICG is also useful in delineating the abnormal aneurysmal outpouchings of the inner choroidal vascular network seen in idiopathic polypoidal choroidal vasculopathy and the focal areas of choroidal hyperpermeability in central serous chorioretinopathy, in differentiating abnormal vasculature in intraocular tumours, and in distinguishing the abnormal fluorescence patterns seen in choroidal inflammatory conditions such as serpiginous choroidopathy, acute multifocal placoid pigment epitheliopathy (AMPPE), multiple evanescent white dot syndrome (MEWDS), birdshot retinochoroidopathy, and multifocal choroiditis. Researchers will likely continue to study ICG as a means of evaluating choroidal circulation in normal and diseased states.

11. TFTTT

List of advantages of OCT-Angiography over IVFA;

– fast (scans take few seconds)
– more user-friendly
– non-invasive
– 3-D images possible
– detailed images at capillary-level blood flow in the retina and choroid
– no dye used. —Red blood cells motion used as contrast
– no need to take images at regular intervals over 10 minutes
– no dye leakage and staining which can hide pathology
– unlike IVFA where early transit of dye can only be captured in one eye at one go, OCT-Angiography can capture both eyes at your comfort
– separate layers easily identified i.e. retinal and choroidal capillary networks
– can identify pathology to early to see clinically.

12. TFTFF

B-scan, or brightness scan, is another method used for ocular assessment via ultrasound. It can be performed directly on the anaesthetised eye. In cases of trauma or in children, B-scan can be performed over the eyelid with coupling jelly. Measurements derived from B-scan include visualisation of the lesion, including anatomic location, shape, borders, and size. It can be used for a detection of a wide-range of pathological structures, including retinal or choroidal detachment, foreign bodies, calcium, and tumours. Echoes in B-scan are converted to dots with brightness intensity that is proportional to the echo amplitude. For example, high amplitude echoes appear as hyper-echoic (white), and absent echoes appear black (anechoic). It is especially useful in imaging of tumours of the anterior orbit, myositis with associated EOM tendon thickening, and visualisation of the superior ophthalmic vein in carotid cavernous fistulas. Similar to A-scan, high gain results in good sensitivity, but poor resolution. It is essential that lesions are centred in the image to obtain the best quality possible.

13. TFTTF

a-wave: initial corneal-negative deflection, derived from the cones and rods of the outer photoreceptor layers
b-wave: corneal-positive deflection; derived from the inner retina, predominantly Muller and ON-bipolar cells

c-wave: derived from the retinal pigment epithelium and photoreceptors
d-wave: off bipolar cells.

Dark adapted Oscillatory potentials: Responses primarily from the amacrine cells/inner retina.

The electrooculogram (EOG) is used to diagnose early Best's disease not the ERG.

14. TFFTF

The resting potential for EOG in normal subject is 6 mV. It is abnormal in disease of RPE. The Arden index is the ratio of light rise to dark trough and in normal subject is more than 165%

Electrooculography (EOG) is a technique for measuring the corneo-retinal standing potential that exists between the front and the back of the human eye. The resulting signal is called the electrooculogram. Primary applications are in ophthalmological diagnosis and in recording eye movements. Unlike the electroretinogram, the EOG does not measure response to individual visual stimuli.

To measure eye movement, pairs of electrodes are typically placed either above and below the eye or to the left and right of the eye. If the eye moves from centre position toward one of the two electrodes, this electrode "sees" the positive side of the retina and the opposite electrode "sees" the negative side of the retina. Consequently, a potential difference occurs between the electrodes. Assuming that the resting potential is constant, the recorded potential is a measure of the eye's position.

The EOG is used to assess the function of the pigment epithelium. During dark adaptation, resting potential decreases slightly and reaches a minimum ("dark trough") after several minutes. When light is switched on, a substantial increase of the resting potential occurs ("light peak"), which drops off after a few minutes when the retina adapts to the light. The ratio of the voltages (i.e. *light peak* divided by *dark trough*) is known as the *Arden ratio*. In practice, the measurement is similar to eye movement recordings (see above). The patient is asked to switch eye position repeatedly between two points (alternating looking from centre to the left and from centre to the right). Since these positions are constant, a change in the recorded potential originates from a change in the resting potential.

15. FFTTT

EOG is useful in detecting Best's disease but is normal in adult onset foveomacular dystrophy

ERG is abnormal in carriers of X-linked retinitis pigmentosa and is diagnostic in Leber's congenital amaurosis

The ERG in Stargardt's disease is variable and is therefore not useful for diagnosis.

A carrier of choroideremia has normal ERG despite changes in the peripheral retina

16. TTTTT

Disease and full-field ERG:

Vitamin A deficiency—Marked rod dysfunction and elevated threshold of rods and cones on dark adaptation

Cancer associated retinopathy (CAR)—Significantly reduced a-wave and b-wave amplitudes

Retinitis pigmentosa—Minimal or sub-normal a- and b-wave amplitudes (response primarily from cone system)

Best Vitelliform Macular Dystrophy—Normal ERG responses with an abnormal EOG

Gyrate Atrophy—Significantly reduced or extinguished rod and cone responses

Carotid Artery Occlusion—Reduced b-wave greater than a-wave amplitudes depending on extent and severity of occlusion

Thioridazine—Decreased photopic and scotopic a- and b-wave responses depending on degree of fundus changes

Carotid Artery Occlusion—Reduced b-wave greater than a-wave amplitudes depending on extent and severity of occlusion

Hypertension and Arteriosclerosis—Initially reduced oscillatory potentials followed by reduced a- and b-wave amplitudes

Chloroquine and Hydroxychloroquine toxicity—Normal ERG responses unless presence of advanced retinopathy; cone function initially more affected than rod function.

References

1. Kenneth Walker H, Dallas Hall W, Willis Hurst J. The funduscopic examination. In: Schneiderman H, editor. Clinical methods: the history, physical, and laboratory examinations, 3rd ed. Boston: Butterworths; 1990. Chapter 117.
2. https://www.aao.org/eyenet/article/new-views-of-retina-with-oct-angiography.
3. Kunimoto D, Kunal K, Mary M. The Wills eye manual: office and emergency room diagnosis and treatment of eye disease, 4th ed. Philadelphia, PA: Lippincott Williams & Wilkins; 2004. p. 365. ISBN 978-0781742078.
4. Manfred Spitznas: Understanding fluorescein angiography = Fluoreszeinangiografie verstehen. (German, English, Spanish). Berlin, Heidelberg, New York: Springer; 2006, ISBN 978-3-540-30060-1.
5. Chaudhari HD, Thakkar GN, Gandhi VS, Darji PJ, Banker HK, Rajwadi H. Role of Ultrasonography in evaluation of orbital lesions. Gujarat Med. J. 2013;68(2):73.
6. Blaivas M, Theodoro D, Sierzenski PR. A study of bedside ocular ultrasonography in the emergency department. Acad Emerg Med. 2002;9(8):791–9.
7. Electrophysiologic Testing in Disorders of the Retina, Optic Nerve, and Visual Pathway (Pearls Series) by Gerald Allen Fishman M.D. Publication Date: January 2, 2001 | ISBN-10: 1560551984 | ISBN-13: 978-1560551980 | Edition: 2.
8. Definition of indocyanine green, National Cancer Institute. https://www.cancer.gov/publications/dictionaries/cancer-drug/def/indocyanine-green-solution.
9. Alander JT, Kaartinen I, Laakso A, Pätilä T, Spillmann T, Tuchin VV, Venermo M, Välisuo P. A review of indocyanine green fluorescent imaging in surgery. Int. J. Biomed. Imag. 2012:940585. https://doi.org/10.1155/2012/940585. PMC 3346977. PMID 22577366.

Chapter 3
Retinal Vascular Disease

1. Diabetic Retinopathy is associated with [1];

   (a) basement membrane thickening
   (b) pericyte loss
   (c) vascular remodelling in later stages
   (d) endothelial barrier decompensation
   (e) extensive serum leakage leading to retinal oedema.

2. Features of proliferative diabetic retinopathy [2];

   (a) associated with capillary non-perfusion
   (b) associated with decreasing levels of VEGF
   (c) treatment is aimed at controlling ischaemia
   (d) anti-VEGFs are the mainstay treatment
   (e) intravitreal steroids do not have any role in the treatment of PDR.

3. Diabetic macular oedema (DMO) [3–5];

   (a) caused by a breakdown of the blood-retina barrier
   (b) associated with hard exudates
   (c) all DMO is associated with vision loss
   (d) occurs only in late stages of PDR
   (e) IVFA is ideal to study the breakdown of the blood-retina barrier.

4. Hypertensive retinopathy is characterised by [6, 7]:

   (a) vitreous haemorrhage
   (b) arteriolar constriction
   (c) superficial flame-shaped haemorrhages early on the disease

© Springer Nature Switzerland AG 2020
M. J. Gouder, *The Retina*, https://doi.org/10.1007/978-3-030-48591-7_3

    (d) optic disc oedema

    (e) flame-shaped haemorrhages.

5. Hypertensive choroidopathy;

    (a) associated with pre-eclampsia

    (b) commoner in older patients

    (c) Elschnig spots and Siegrist streaks are a feature

    (d) can cause RPE detachments

    (e) associated with bilateral rhegmatogenous retinal detachments.

6. Hypertensive optic neuropathy [8];

    (a) common in benign systemic hypertension

    (b) features flame-shaped haemorrhages

    (c) can mimic radiation retinopathy

    (d) can be associated with a macular star

    (e) is reversible.

7. Risk factors in central retinal vein occlusion [9];

    (a) smoking

    (b) middle-age

    (c) glaucoma

    (d) leukaemia

    (e) systemic hypertension.

8. Amaurosis fugax [10];

    (a) transient binocular loss of vision

    (b) painful

    (c) mostly of embolic origin

    (d) can be associated with a transient ischaemic attack

    (e) should not be investigated.

9. In Central Retinal Artery Occlusion (CRAO):

    (a) is always painless

    (b) visual acuity is always severely low

    (c) RAPD is common

    (d) clinically featured with a 'cherry-red spot'

    (e) IVFA shows delayed arterial filling.

10. Hard exudates:

   (a) composed of lipid and lipoprotein
   (b) found in the inner plexiform layer
   (c) common in uveitis
   (d) commonly found on top of the retinal vessels
   (e) a macular star is commonly associated with infective papillitis.

1   Answers

   1. TTFTT
   2. TFTTF
   3. TTFFT
   4. FTFTT
   5. TFTTF
   6. FTTTF
   7. TFTTT
   8. TFTTT
   9. FFTTT
  10. TFFFT.

2   Answers in Detail

1. TTFTT

Hyperglycaemia leads to:

 – inflammatory oxidative stress
 – advanced glycation end-products
 – Protein C pathway disruption.

All the above leads to endothelial cell damage and pericyte loss. There is increased platelet and erythrocyte aggregation and adhesion which is compounded by defective fibrinolysis. Vascular remodelling can even be seen in early stages associated with background diabetic retinopathy as seen on recent advances in OCT angiography. The hallmark of diabetic retinopathy (DR) is vascular changes involving different retinal layers. OCTA enables detection of retinal vascular abnormalities including areas of capillary non-perfusion, changes in foveal avascular zone (FAZ), and impairment of the choriocapillaris (CC) flow in diabetics with no apparent DR. OCTA may be able not only to detect diabetic eyes at a higher risk of retinopathy but also to screen for diabetes mellitus (DM) even before systemic diagnosis is made. OCTA demonstrates that retinal vascular pathology including clustered capillaries, dilated capillary segments, tortuous capillaries, regions of capillary dropout, reduced capillary density, abnormal capillary loops, and FAZ enlargement are evident in both non-proliferative and proliferative diabetic retinopathy.

2. TFTTF

With worsening diabetic retinopathy both capillary damage and non-perfusion become prominent leading to worsening ischaemia which in turn leads to the release of pro-angiogenic factors like vascular endothelial growth factors. This is followed by neovascularisation at the disc (NVD), iris (NVI) and elsewhere on the retina (NVE). Treatment is based on the idea that reperfusion may help the damaged ischaemic retina. Anti-VEGF treatment is highly effective in the treatment of recently diagnosed but also in chronic disease. Steroids are not used as a primary treatment of PDR but are effective in the treatment of diabetic macular oedema (DMO).

3. TTFFT

Diabetic macular oedema is the most common cause of visual loss in those with diabetic retinopathy and is increasing in prevalence globally. The prevalence of DME in patients with diabetic retinopathy is 2.7–11% and it depends on the type of diabetes and the duration of the disease, but for both types 1 and 2 after 25-years duration, it approximates 30%. Systemic factors associated with DM include longer duration of diabetes, higher systolic blood pressure, and higher haemoglobin A1c.

Hyperglycaemia causes the breakdown of the blood-retina barrier leading to leakage from retinal vessels and once there is retinal thickening it is clearly seen on OCT macular scans. The thickening can also be associated with leaked plasma lipoproteins causing the characteristic associated hard exudates. If the leakage and thickening is central then vision loss is very evident but if the leakage and thickening is off-centre or eccentric one might still enjoy good vision. Even eyes with mild non-proliferative diabetic retinopathy (NPDR) can have a substantial vision loss from DMO.

4. FTFTT

In hypertensive retinopathy there are arteriolar changes, such as generalised arteriolar narrowing, focal arteriolar narrowing, arteriovenous nicking, changes in the arteriolar wall (arteriosclerosis) and abnormalities at points where arterioles and venules cross. Manifestations of these changes include Copper wire arterioles where the central light reflex occupies most of the width of the arteriole and Silver wire arterioles where the central light reflex occupies all of the width of the arteriole, and "arterio-venous (AV) nicking" or "AV nipping", due to venous constriction and banking.

In advanced retinopathy lesions one can find signs such as microaneurysms, blot haemorrhages and/or flame haemorrhages, ischemic changes (e.g. "cotton wool spots"), hard exudates and in severe cases swelling of the optic disc (optic disc edema), a ring of exudates around the retina called a "macular star" and visual acuity loss—typically due to macular involvement.

Mild signs of hypertensive retinopathy can be seen quite frequently in normal people (3–14% of adult individuals aged ≥ 40 years), even without hypertension.

Hypertensive retinopathy is commonly considered a diagnostic feature of a hypertensive emergency although it is not invariably present.

5. TFTTF

Features of hypertensive choroidopathy include:

- occurs in young patients with a hypertensive crisis
- found in pre-eclampsia, eclampsia, phaechromocytoma, renal hypertension
- Elschnig spots—areas of hyperpigmentation surrounded by hypo-pigmented margin caused by lobular choroidal non-perfusion
- Siegrist streaks—linear hyperpigmentation following the meridional course of choroidal arteries
- focal RPE detachments. Although they are usually indicative of fibrinoid necrosis associated with malignant hypertension, Siegrist streaks also occur in patients with temporal arteritis
- bilateral exudative retinal detachments (in pregnancy may resolve on its own after birth).

6. FTTTF

Hypertensive optic neuropathy:

Associated with malignant uncontrolled acute hypertension and is characterised by:

- flame-shaped haemorrhages around the optic disc
- blurred Optic nerve head margins
- peripapillary venous stasis
- macular exudates
- reversible on controlling the hypertension.

Differential diagnosis of Hypertensive Optic Neuropathy;

- central retinal vein occlusion (CRVO)
- anterior ischaemic optic neuropathy (AION)
- diabetic papillopathy
- neuroretinitis
- radiation papillopathy.

7. TFTTT

- advanced age
- male gender

- smoking
- arteriosclerosis
- hypertension
- diabetes mellitus
- hyperlipidaemia
- vascular cerebral stroke
- blood hyperviscosity
- thrombophilia
- race.

A strong risk factor for retinal vein occlusion (RVO) is the metabolic syndrome (hypertension, diabetes mellitus, and hyperlipidaemia). Also individuals with end-organ damage caused by diabetes mellitus and hypertension have greatly increased risk for RVO. Socioeconomic status seems to be a risk factor too. American blacks are more often diagnosed with RVO than non-Hispanic whites. Females are, according to some studies, at lower risk than men. The role of throm-bophilic risk factors in RVO is still controversial. Congenital thrombophilic dis-eases like factor V Leiden mutation, hyperhomocysteinaemia and anticardiolipin antibodies increase the risk of RVO. Cigarette smoking also increases the risk of RVO as do systemic inflammatory conditions like vasculitis and Behcet disease. Ophthalmic risk factors for RVO are ocular hypertension and glaucoma, higher ocular perfusion pressure, and changes in the retinal arteries.

8. TFTTT

Amaurosis fugax from the Greek *amaurosis* meaning *darkening*, *dark*, or *obscure and* Latin *fugax* meaning *fleeting*) is a painless temporary loss of vision in one or both eyes (less common). Amaurosis fugax which is commonly defined as a painless monocular vision loss is usually associated with embolic phenomena. The vision loss can last for a few minutes and can be associated with systemic symp-toms of TIA. The patient should be thoroughly investigated as there is a risk of stroke. Loss of vision is usually fast and recovery is usually slower.

9. FFTTT

CRAO is characterised by profound loss of vision which is usually painless. 80% of affected individuals will end up with a final visual acuity of counting fingers or worse. However if the cilioretinal artery is spared, vision may be only slightly decreased because of preservation of the cilioretinal artery which supplies the macular area. Complete loss of vision can be an indication that the ophthalmic artery is actually embolised localising the pathology more posteriorly. The con-dition is painful if it is associated with Giant Cell Arteritis. The choroidal vas-culature is intact in CRAO and the bright orange reflex from the healthy choroid can stand out at the macular area. This is called a 'cherry red spot' which usually subsides later on. Delayed arterial filling in IVFA is expected because the cen-tral retinal artery is blocked. However this can be variable. Retinal oedema can cause a blocking defect hence it will look hypofluorescent. IVFA is excellent to demonstrate a patent cilioretinal artery in those with some degree of visual preservation. The incidence of CRAO is approximately 1–2 in 100,000 with a male predominance and mean age of 60–65 years.

10. TFFFT

Hard exudates are well-circumscribed and can be found deep to the retinal vessels in the outer plexiform layer and not the inner layer. Hard exudates are commonly associated with diabetic retinopathy but also with optic nerve pathology such as infarction and inflammation leading to the formation of a macular star. Sometimes macular stars are asymptomatic and when the star is more accentuated nasally it is more associated with primary optic nerve pathology. Hard exudates that assume a star appearance is usually because the lipids accumulates in Henle's layer around the macula.

References

1. J Ophthalmic Vis Res. 2018 Oct-Dec; 13(4): 487–497. https://doi.org/10.4103/jovr. jovr_57_18 PMCID: PMC6210870 PMID: 30479720 An Update on Optical Coherence Tomography Angiography in Diabetic Retinopathy Joobin Khadamy, MD, Kaveh Abri Aghdam, MD, PhD, and Khalil Ghasemi Falavarjani, MD.
2. Antonetti DA, Klein R, Gardner TW. Diabetic retinopathy. N Engl J Med. 2012;366(13):1227–39. https://doi.org/10.1056/nejmra1005073.
3. Xie XW, Xu L, Wang YX, Jonas JB. Prevalence and associated factors of diabetic retinopathy. The Beijing Eye Study 2006. Graefes Arch Clin Exp Ophthalmol. 2008;246(11):1519–26.
4. Wong TY, Klein R, Islam FM, Cotch MF, Folsom AR, Klein BE, Sharrett AR, Shea S. Diabetic retinopathy in a multi-ethnic cohort in the United States. Am J Ophthalmol. 2006;141(3):446–55.
5. Browning DJ, Stewart MW, Lee C. Diabetic macular edema: evidence-based management. Indian J Ophthalmol. 2018;66(12): 1736–1750. https://doi.org/10.4103/ijo.ijo_1240_18.
6. Bhargava M, Ikram MK, Wong TY. How does hypertension affect your eyes? J Human Hypertens. 2011;26(2).
7. Yanoff M, Duker JS. Ophthalmology. Elsevier Health Sciences; 2009. ISBN 978-0323043328.
8. Kovach JL. Hypertensive optic neuropathy and choroidopathy in an 18-year-old woman with renal failure. Retin Cases Brief Rep. 2010;4(2):187–9. https://doi.org/10.1097/icb.0b013e31819d2641.
9. Kolar P. Risk factors for central and branch retinal vein occlusion: a meta-analysis of published clinical data. J Ophthalmol. 2014;2014:724780. https://doi.org/10.1155/2014/724780. Epub 2014 Jun.
10. Fisher CM. 'Transient monocular blindness' versus 'amaurosis fugax'. Neurology. 1989;39(12):1622–4. https://doi.org/10.1212/wnl.39.12.1622. PMID 2685658.

Chapter 4
Retinal Degeneration and Dystrophies

1. Stargardt Disease [1, 2]:

   (a) is mainly an autosomal recessive disease
   (b) affects mainly peripheral vision
   (c) is a progressive disease leading to legal blindness
   (d) there is abnormal metabolism of Vitamin A and E
   (e) is very common.

2. Best's Disease [3]:

   (a) is autosomal recessive
   (b) there is a normal EOG and abnormal ERG
   (c) there is an abnormal EOG and a normal ERG
   (d) is associated with poor vision in the early stages
   (e) CNV development is sometimes seen.

3. Retinitis Pigmentosa [4];

   (a) autosomal recessive
   (b) most common hereditary fundus dystrophy
   (c) prevalence of approximately 1 in 50,000
   (d) autosomal dominant
   (e) X-linked recessive.

4. Retinitis pigmentosa [5];

   (a) predominantly affects rod photoreceptors
   (b) initially affects cone photoreceptors
   (c) ERG amplitude is reduced early on in the disease

© Springer Nature Switzerland AG 2020
M. J. Gouder, *The Retina*, https://doi.org/10.1007/978-3-030-48591-7_4

(d) ERG changes occur after retinal changes are visible
(e) can mimic syphilitic pigmentary retinopathy.

5. Familial dominant drusen (Doyne honeycomb choroiditis) [6];

   (a) also known as malattia leventinese
   (b) gene mutation in EFEMP1
   (c) similar fundus to ARMD
   (d) abnormal ERG snd EOG
   (e) carries a very good visual prognosis.

6. Stickler syndrome [7];

   (a) increased risk of retinal detachment
   (b) patients have mid-facial hypoplasia
   (c) Stickler syndrome type 4 is non-ocular
   (d) associated with myopia
   (e) associated with vitreous changes.

7. Familial exudative vitreoretinoapthy (FEVR) [8];

   (a) similar picture to retinopathy of prematurity
   (b) carries a very good visual prognosis
   (c) commonly autosomal dominant
   (d) associated with hyperopia
   (e) can be exudative.

8. Pattern dystrophy [9];

   (a) autosomal dominant
   (b) clinical picture similar to ARMD
   (c) very progressive disease
   (d) patients lose vision early on the disease
   (e) caused by lipofuscin accumulation.

9. Juvenile X-linked retinoschisis [10, 11];

   (a) occurs almost exclusively in males
   (b) characterised by symmetric bilateral macular schisis
   (c) there is schisis of the peripheral retina in all cases
   (d) visual acuity often deteriorates during the first and second decades of life
   (e) associated with the Mizuo phenomenon.

10. Choroideremia [12, 13];

    (a) autosomal recessive
    (b) nyctalopia
    (c) initially can mimic RP
    (d) poor visual prognosis
    (e) carriers have normal fundi.

11. Peripheral retinal changes;

    (a) peripheral cystoid degeneration is common in adulthood
    (b) peripheral drusen is similar to drusen found in the posterior pole
    (c) pavingstone degeneration is very rare
    (d) 'white without pressure' (WWOP) is associated with giant retinal tears
        (GRT)
    (e) reticular degeneration is frequently associated with retinal detachment.

1   Answers

    1. TFTFF
    2. FFTFT
    3. TTFTT
    4. TFTFT
    5. TTTFF
    6. TTFTT
    7. TFTFT
    8. TTFFT
    9. TTFTT
   10. FTTTF
   11. TTFTF.

2   Answers in Detail

1. TFTFF

Stargardt disease is the most common inherited single-gene retinal disease. It is commonly autosomal recessive (ABCA4 gene) and very rarely autosomal dominant (ELOVL4 or PROM1 gene). It is a form of 'accelerated' macular degeneration occurring earlier in childhood and continues to progress in adulthood leading to legal blindness. The median age of onset: ~17 years old, very commonly before age 20.

The fundus is typically full of white flecks with central macular atrophy in later stages (fundus flavimaculatus). The gene is responsible for vitamin A transport between the photoreceptors and RPE. Vitamin E is not involved. The disease is rare and is considered to be one of the 'orphan diseases' which means not much pharmaceutical companies are ready to invest in research. There is no treatment but three strategies are recommended for potential harm reduction: reducing retinal exposure to damaging ultraviolet light, avoiding foods rich in Vitamin A with the hope of lowering lipofuscin accumulation and maintaining good general health and diet.

2. FFTFT

Best disease is an AD disease associated with an abnormal BEST1 gene which produces a dysfunctional bestrophin gene which leads to the accumulation of lipofuscin and fluid under the macula giving it an egg yolk appearance (Vitelliform coming from Latin *vitellus* meaning egg yolk).

Although it is an autosomal dominant condition, many affected people, however, have no history of the disorder in their family and only a small number of affected families have been reported. This is because the penetrance of the condition is incomplete; therefore, it is possible for an individual to have a copy of the mutant allele and not display the VMD phenotype. The ratio of males to females is approximately 1:1.

There is an abnormal EOG with an Arden ratio of < 1.5 (normal > 1.5 preferably > 1.85). Visual acuity and metamorphopsia usually occur very later in the 'scrambled egg stage' and also when CNV develops (in ~ 20% of cases). An adult form exists called Adult Vitelliform Macular degeneration which usually shows smaller lesions and a normal EOG.

3. TTFTT

RP is the most common hereditary fundus dystrophy with a prevalence of 1 in 5000. The age of onset, progression rate, eventual visual loss and associated ocular features are frequently associated with the mode of inheritance. Retinitis pigmentosa can be sporadic or inherited. Mutations of the rhodopsin gene will lead to the retinal clinical features of retinitis pigmentosa. The sporadic form has a very good prognosis but the best prognosis is found if RP is inherited in the AD way.

In *autosomal recessive inheritance*, the disease can be severe. It takes two copies of the mutant gene to give rise to the disorder. An individual with a recessive gene mutation is known as a carrier. When two carriers have a child, there is a:

- 1 in 4 chance the child will have the disorder
- 1 in 2 chance the child will be a carrier
- 1 in 4 chance the child will neither have the disorder nor be a carrier.

In autosomal dominant inheritance, it takes just one copy of the gene with a disorder-causing mutation to bring about the disorder. When a parent has a dominant gene mutation, there is a 1 in 2 chance that any children will inherit this mutation and the disorder.

X-linked Inheritance (least common but most severe)

In this form of inheritance, mothers carry the mutated gene on one of their X chromosomes and pass it to their sons. Because females have two X chromosomes, the effect of a mutation on one X chromosome is offset by the normal gene on the other X chromosome. If a mother is a carrier of an X-linked disorder there is a:

- 1 in 2 chance of having a son with the disorder
- 1 in 2 chance of having a daughter who is a carrier.

4. TFTFT

Retinitis pigmentosa predominantly affects rod photoreceptors followed by degeneration of cone photoreceptors. ERG is extinguished early in the disease and before there are obvious clinical retinal pigmentary changes. ERG is extinguished in severe cases without detectable rod or cone responses to white light. Multifocal ERG may provide more specific information.

EOG is subnormal in RP with absence of light rise. Retinitis pigments can be syndromic such as in Usher syndrome where patients also have hearing loss. It can mimic syphilitic retinopathy and congenital rubella syndrome where patients will also feature hearing loss.

Usher syndrome is a condition characterised by partial or total hearing loss and vision loss that worsens over time. The hearing loss is classified as sensorineural, which means that it is caused by abnormalities of the inner ear.

5. TTTFF

Doyne honeycomb dystrophy:

Most cases of Doyne honeycomb dystrophy are caused by a mutation on a single gene called EFEMP1. This causes the gene to 'fold' a protein wrongly, and stops it breaking down as it should. The protein then builds up to create 'drusen' inside the eye tissue and stops nutrients getting from blood vessels to the light-sensing cells that need them. As the cells waste and die, sight is lost.

Doyne honeycomb dystrophy is an autosomal dominant condition.

Symptoms:

- metamorphosis
- blurred vision
- scotomas
- light adaptation issues.

The symptoms are caused by drusen forming near the macula, and at the point where the optic nerve enters the eye. The drusen start small and gradually grow together, forming a honeycomb pattern.

It usually develops in early-to-mid adulthood, although occasionally teenagers are affected. Once the drusen appear, people gradually lose their central vision, although peripheral side vision is not affected. Some people have more rapid sight loss caused by new blood vessels growing behind the macula. In such cases anti-VEGF can be used with limited improvement expected.

6. TTFTT

Stickler syndrome is also called hereditary arthro-ophthalmopathy and is actually a group of hereditary group of disorders affecting collagen type II and X. It is the most common inherited cause of retinal detachment in children. Typically there is a radial lattice type retinal changes associated with RPE hyperplasia Table 4.1.

There is a fourth variant of Stickler syndrome (STL4) with the genetic defect COL9A1. This is the recessive variant.

Pierre Robin sequence;

- micrognathia (abnormally small jaw or mandible
- cleft palate
- glossoptosis resulting in airway obstruction caused by backwards displacement of the tongue base
- bifid uvula
- Mild spondylo-epiphyseal dysplasia
- joint hypermobility
- early-onset osteoarthritis.

Table 4.1 Types of stickler syndrome

	Type I (STL1)	Type II (STL2)	Type III (STL3)
Ocular	Myopia Membranous vitre-ous (optically-empty vitreous) Retrolenticular membrane Circumferential equatorial membranes that extend a short way into the vitreous cavity Cataract Retinal detachment Blindness	Congenital non-progressive high myopia Beaded/fibrillary vitreous Cataract	No ocular symptoms
Craniofacial	Cleft palate Pierre-Robin sequence	Cleft palate Pierre-Robin sequence	Mid-facial hypoplasia and palatal abnormalities
Auditory	Mild-to-moderate hearing loss	Early-onset sensorineural hearing loss, mild to moderate	Hearing loss
Articular	Early onset osteoarthritis, joint hyper mobility, spondylo-epiphyseal dysplasia		Early onset osteoarthritis, short stature
Genetics	COL2A1 (75% of stickler cases)	COL11A1	COL11A2

7. TFTFT

In FEVR there is failure of retinal vascularisation (mainly temporal) which gives a clinical picture similar to retinopathy of prematurity but appearing in children who had been born full-term with normal birthweight.

FEVR is usually bilateral and asymmetric. It can present at any age, and the mean age of presentation is 6 years. It has very poor visual prognosis especially if the disease occurs early and is aggressive. Mainly inherited in an autosomal dominant fashion and very commonly associated with high myopia.

The main hallmark of FEVR is an avascular peripheral retina with subsequent dragging of the vessels, with or without retinal folds, as well as preretinal, intraretinal, or subretinal exudation.

Retinal detachment is common and can be exudative, tractional or rhegmatogenous.

Wide-field IVFA shows:

- peripheral retinal non-perfusion
- vessel pruning
- avascularity
- neovascularization
- straightening of vessels
- peripheral vascular anastomoses.

Pre-retinal fibrovascular proliferation is also a feature. It is associated with neovascular glaucoma.

8. TTFFT

Pattern dystrophy is the umbrella term for a group of retinal conditions in which a build-up of waste material called lipofuscin causes damage to tissues in the eye. Different dystrophies cause different patterns of damage, which might look like egg yolks, butterflies or knotted fishing nets. People will usually have symptoms in both eyes, and may have a different pattern of damage in each. The symptoms of pattern dystrophy are similar to age-related macular degeneration (ARM(D), but tend to be less severe. Despite some blurring of vision and loss of fine detail, people are usually able to drive and read the newspaper. Often, the lipofuscin deposits are picked up during a regular eye test before the patient notices any sight loss.

Although symptoms do get worse, this usually happens very slowly, over 20–30 years. Around 15% of people develop new, leaky blood vessels in their eye tissue (like wet AMD). A similar proportion find that patches of the light-sensing cells in their retina start to die off due to geographic atrophy (also a symptom of dry AMD). This usually happens in people aged over 60.

9. TTFTT

X-linked Retinoschisis, or X-Linked Juvenile Retinoschisis is a rare congenital malformation of the retina caused by mutations in the *RS1* gene, which encodes retinoschisin, a protein involved in intercellular adhesion and likely retinal cellular organisation. X-Linked juvenile retinoschisis occurs in males and typically present with bilateral reduced visual acuity 6/36–6/60. There are areas of schisis characterised by splitting of the nerve fibre layer of the retina. The macula assumes a spoke-wheel pattern. There is schisis of the peripheral retina, predominantly inferotemporally, in approximately 50% of individuals. The associated elevation of the surface layer of the retina into the vitreous has been described as "vitreous veils". Sometimes the Mizuo phenomenon occurs, a colour change in the retina after dark adaptation with the onset of light. OCT reveals characteristic signs such as foveal schisis and retinal thinning.

10. FTTTF

This is an X-linked inherited condition (rarely other inheritance patterns) affecting both eyes. The majority of the patients seen will be male. Most cases seen in the examination are either established or end-stage choideremia.

In established cases, there is atrophy of the retinal pigment epithelium and choroid with exposure of the sclera and large choroidal blood vessels. The condition usually starts in the equator and spread centrally and peripherally. There are usually pigmentary changes on the fundus giving it a 'salt and pepper' appearance.

In advanced cases, the fundus appears 'white-out' with total choroidal atrophy and exposure of the sclera.

In the female carrier the most common feature is pigmentary changes in the mid-periphery. There may also be patchy degeneration of the RPE and choroid with drusenoid deposition.

The visual prognosis is poor and the peripheral visual field is affected early on life i.e. around the teenage years. Nyctalopia is prominent. However central visual field is usually retained until later 50 s.

Differential diagnosis of choideremia;

- Serpiginous choroidopathy
- Punctuate Inner Choroidopathy (PIC)
- Gyrate atrophy
- Central areolar sclerosis
- Generalised choroidal atrophy.

11. TTFTF

Peripheral cystoid degeneration makes the retina looks thicker and less transparent and is common in adulthood. Peripheral drusen is also common in adulthood and the drusenoid material is similar to drusen found in the posterior pole around the macula. It is sometimes pigmented. Pavingstone degeneration is associated with focal chorioretinal atrophy and more common in the inferior peripheral fundus and present in a quarter of adult eyes. 'White without pressure' has the same appearance as 'white with pressure' (WWP) but is present without scleral indentation. It is associated with an anomalous relatively strong condensed vitreous and this increases the risk of giant retinal tears forming along its posterior border. This is preferably lasered prophylactically. Reticular degeneration is also known as honeycomb degeneration and is also associated with the ageing retina and consists of pigmentation occurring along the peripheral retinal vessels. This is not usually pathologic.

References

1. Clinical Characteristics and Current Therapies for Inherited Retinal Degenerations Jose. Alain Sahel.
2. Stargardt disease/Fundus flavimaculatus. EyeWiki. eyewiki.aao.org.
3. MacDonald IM, Lee T. Best vitelliform macular dystrophy. In: Adam MP, Ardinger HH, Pagon RA, Wallace SE, Bean LJ, Stephens K, Amemiya A, MacDonald IM, Lee T, editors. Gene reviews. Seattle, WA: University of Washington, Seattle; 2003.
4. Facts About Retinitis Pigmentosa. National Eye Institute; May 2014.
5. Aparisi MJ, Aller E, Fuster-García C, García-García G, Rodrigo R, Vázquez-Manrique RP, Blanco-Kelly F, Ayuso C, Roux AF, Jaijo T, Millán JM. Targeted next generation sequencing for molecular diagnosis of Usher syndrome. Orphanet J Rare Dis. 2014;18(9):168. https://doi.org/10.1186/s13023-014-0168-7.
6. https://www.macularsociety.org/doyne-honeycomb-dystrophy.
7. Liberfarb RM, Levy HP, Rose PS, Wilki DJ, Davis J, Balog JZ, Griffith AJ, Szymko-Bennett YM, Johnston JJ, Francomano CA, Tsilou E, Rubin BI. The Stickler syndrome: genotype/phenotype correlation in 10 families with Stickler syndrome resulting from seven mutations in the type II collagen gene locus COL2A1. Genet Med. 2003;5(1):21–7. https://doi.org/10.1097/00125817-200301000-00004. PMID 12544472.
8. Criswick VG, Schepens CL. Familial exudative vitreoretinopathy. Am J Ophthalmol. 1969;68(4):578–94. http://retinatoday.com/2013/03/update-on-fevr-diagnosis-management-and-treatment/.
9. Alkuraya H, Zhang K. Pattern dystrophy of the retinal pigment epithelium. https://www.retinalphysician.com/issues/2010/may-2010/peer-reviewed-pattern-dystrophy-of-the-retinal-pi.
10. Sieving PA, MacDonald IM, Chan S. X-Linked juvenile retinoschisis. https://ghr.nlm.nih.gov/condition/x-linked-juvenile-retinoschisis.
11. Sikkink SK, Biswas S, Parry NRA, Stanga PE, Trump D. X-linked retinoschisis: an update. J Med Genet. 2007;44(4):225–32.
12. Pennesi ME, Birch DG, Duncan JL, Bennett J, Girach A. Choroideremia: retinal degeneration with an unmet need. Retina. 2019. https://doi.org/10.1097/iae.0000000000002553.
13. http://www.mrcophth.com/macula/choroideremia.html.

Chapter 5
Disorders of the Macula

1. CATT study [1];

   (a) compared ranibizumab and bevacizumab
   (b) the results show no major difference in VA outcome between the above two
   (c) the study compared the outcome of the above two when given bimonthly and prn
   (d) bevacizumab had less systemic side effects than ranibizumab
   (e) ranibizumab produced greater decrease in macular thickness.

2. Bevacizumab [2];

   (a) used in the treatment of colon cancer
   (b) used in the treatment of glioblastoma
   (c) is a monoclonal antibody
   (d) is more expensive than ranibizumab
   (e) inhibits Vascular Endothelial Growth factor A (VEGF-A).

3. Risk factors for age-related macular degeneration (ARMD);

   (a) family history
   (b) smoking
   (c) systemic hypotension
   (d) obesity
   (e) aspirin.

4. The incidence of Central Serous Retinopathy (CSR) is higher in [3];

   (a) young females
   (b) Pickwickian syndrome

© Springer Nature Switzerland AG 2020
M. J. Gouder, *The Retina*, https://doi.org/10.1007/978-3-030-48591-7_5

(c) Cushing syndrome
(d) pregnancy
(e) use of non-steroidal anti-inflammatory medications (NSAIDs).

5. Treatment of CSR [4–6]:

   (a) argon laser to the leakage site
   (b) lifestyle changes
   (c) spironolactone
   (d) epleronone
   (e) aspirin.

6. Cystoid Macular Oedema [7];

   (a) involves fluid accumulation in the inner plexiform layer
   (b) can occur in retinitis pigmentosa
   (c) complicated cataract surgery
   (d) associated with the use of brinzolamide drops
   (e) associated with foveal lamellar hole.

7. Angioid Streaks are associated with [8];

   (a) Paget's disease
   (b) breaks in Bruch's membrane
   (c) an intact RPE
   (d) Juvenile xanthogranuloma
   (e) choroidal neovascularization.

8. Solar maculopathy;

   (a) caused exclusively by staring at the sun
   (b) visual acuity loss is permanent
   (c) caused by thermal damage to the retina
   (d) associated with macular oedema
   (e) treated with steroids.

9. Hypotonic maculopathy [9, 10];

   (a) associated with an IOP <6.5 mmHg
   (b) painful, decreased vision
   (c) hyperopic shift
   (d) associated with choroidal folds
   (e) pale optic disc.

10. Degenerative myopic maculopathy is associated with:

    (a) Down's Syndrome
    (b) Pierre-Robin Syndrome
    (c) prematurity
    (d) legal blindness
    (e) posterior staphyloma.

11. Tay-Sachs disease [11];

    (a) autosomal dominant
    (b) commoner in Jewish infants
    (c) causes a generalised neurological deterioration
    (d) life expectancy up to the early 20s
    (e) associated with hearing loss.

1   Answers

   1. TTFFT
   2. TTTFT
   3. TTFTT
   4. FTTTF
   5. FTTTT
   6. FTTFT
   7. TTFFT
   8. FFFTT
   9. TFTTF
  10. TTTTT
  11. FTTFT.

2   Answers in Detail

1. TTFFT

The CATT study (US) compared 2 year results comparing ranibizumab with bevacizumab in a head-to-head study in patients with exudative AMD. The results were presented in the 2012 ARVO meeting. Mean visual acuity results of bevacizumab were equivalent to ranibizumab at both monthly and prn dosing (not bimonthly) however mean gain in vision was greater with monthly injection vs prn injection for both drugs. Bevacizumab, apart from being cheaper, produced more systemic side effects (mainly vascular—myocardial infarction, stroke) than ranibizumab but the relation is uncertain. Ranibizumab does appear to result in a lower risk of stomach and intestinal problems. Ranibizumab produced greater decrease in macular thickness however it also affirmed the effectiveness of off-label bevacizumab in treating neovascular AMD.

2. TTTFT

Ranibizumab is a monoclonal antibody fragment (Fab) created from the same parent mouse antibody as bevacizumab. It is an anti-angiogenic that has been approved to treat the "wet" type of age-related macular degeneration. It inhibits vascular endothelial growth factor A, a mechanism similar to bevacizumab.

Its effectiveness is similar to that of bevacizumab and aflibercept-rates of side effects also appear similar. However, ranibizumab typically costs $2,000 a dose, while the equivalent dose of bevacizumab typically costs $50.

A 2017 systematic review update found that while ranibizumab and bevacizumab provide similar functional outcomes in diabetic macular edema, there is low-certainty evidence suggesting that ranibizumab is more effective in reducing central retinal thickness than bevacizumab.

3. TTFTT

Age remains the most dominant risk factor in developing age-related macular degeneration. Older white individuals have a higher risk than older black individuals. Family history is also important with the risk being three times the normal if a first degree individual has the condition. Smoking doubles the risk. Hypertension, obesity and the lack of intake of antioxidants are also associated with increased risk of this disease. There is some evidence that aspirin increases the risk of ARMD.

4. FTTTF

CSR is a fluid detachment of the macula layers from their supporting tissue. This allows choroidal fluid to leak beneath the retina. The buildup of fluid seems to occur because of small breaks in the retinal pigment epithelium.

CSR is associated with

– high cortisol levels (such as in stress and Cushing syndrome)
– steroid use
– sympathomimetics.
– *Helicobacter pylori*

5. FTTTT

Traditional argon laser is not indicated anymore as there is a huge risk to the fovea. Yellow micro-pulse diode laser is a more common trend nowadays as it is associated with less damage to the fovea. This is also supported by OCT analysis in such cases.

People who have irregular sleep patterns, type A personalities, sleep apnea, or systemic hypertension are more susceptible to CSR. Elevated circulating cortisol and epinephrine affect the auto-regulation of the choroidal circulation. With management of these lifestyle patterns and associated cortisol and epinephrine levels, it has been shown that the fluid associated with CSR can spontaneously resolve. Melatonin has been shown to help regulate sleep in people who have irregular sleep patterns in turn better regulating cortisol and epinephrine levels to manage CSR.

Medications;

Spironolactone is a mineralocorticoid receptor antagonist that has been proven to help reduce the fluid associated with CSR. In a study noted by Acta Ophthalmologica, spironolactone improved visual acuity in CSR patients over the course of 8 weeks.

Epleronone is another mineralocorticoid receptor antagonist that has been proven to reduce the subretinal fluid that is present with CSR. In a study noted in International Journal of Ophthalmology, results showed epleronone decreased the subretinal fluid both horizontally and vertically over time. Though after stopping the medication, the fluid also appeared to return and patients needed further treatment.

Low dosage ibuprofen has been shown to quicken recovery in some cases.

Aspirin also showed some benefit in some patients.

6. FTTFT

Cystoid macular edema (CME) involves fluid accumulation between the outer plexiform layer and inner nuclear layer of the retina secondary to abnormal perifoveal retinal capillary permeability. The oedema is termed "cystoid" as it appears cystic; however, lacking an epithelial coating, it is not truly cystic.

The causes of macular edema are numerous and different causes may be inter-related.

- It is commonly associated with diabetes. Chronic or uncontrolled diabetes type 2 can affect peripheral blood vessels including those of the retina which may leak fluid, blood and occasionally fats into the retina causing it to swell
- Age-related macular degeneration may cause macular edema. As individuals age there may be a natural deterioration in the macula which can lead to the depositing of drusen under the retina sometimes with the formation of abnormal blood vessels
- ERM
- Retinal capillary haemangiomas
- Chronic renal failure
- Cataract surgery—pseudophakic macular edema
- Chronic uveitis and intermediate uveitis
- CRVO, BRVO
- Toxic drug effects: latanoprost, epinephrine, rosiglitazone, timolol and thiazolidinediones
- RP
- Retinoschisis.

If the small fluid cysts coalesce they can form larger cysts and increase the risk of foveal lamellar hole leading to irreversible impairment of central vision.

7. TTFFT

Angioid streaks, also known as Knapp striae, are irregular jagged dehiscences in the mineralised, degenerated, brittle Bruch membrane that typically form alongside force lines exerted by intrinsic and extrinsic ocular muscles that radiate in a centrifugal pattern emanating from the optic disc.

Angioid streaks are often associated with pseudoxanthoma elasticum (PXE), but have been found to occur in conjunction with other disorders, including Paget's disease, Sickle cell disease and Ehlers-Danlos Syndrome. These streaks can have a negative impact on vision due to choroidal neovascularization or choroidal rupture. Also, vision can be impaired if the streaks progress to the fovea and damage the retinal pigment epithelium. Diagnosis mainly clinical, however IVFA shows that the streaks appear hyperfluorescent (window defect) in the early phase.

8. FFFTT

Photic retinopathy, also known as foveomacular retinitis or solar retinopathy, is damage to the eye's retina, particularly the macula, from prolonged exposure to solar radiation or other bright light, e.g., lasers or arc welders. The term includes solar, laser, and welder's retinopathy and is synonymous with retinal phototoxicity. It usually occurs due to staring at the sun like when watching a solar eclipse.

Vision loss (central or paracentral) due to solar retinopathy is typically reversible, lasting for as short as one month to over one year. The fundus changes are variable and usually bilateral with mild cases often show no alteration whilst moderate to severe cases show a foveal yellow spot on the first days after exposure. After a few days it is replaced by a reddish dot often surrounded by pigment.

Permanent holes and lesions are possible; prognosis worsens with dilated pupils or prolonged exposure.

Although it is frequently claimed that the retina is burned by looking at the sun, retinal damage appears to occur primarily due to photochemical injury rather than thermal injury. The temperature rise from looking at the sun with a 3-mm pupil only causes a 4 °C increase in temperature, insufficient to photocoagulate. The energy is still phototoxic: since light promotes oxidation, chemical reactions occur in the exposed tissues with unbonded oxygen molecules. It also appears that central serous retinopathy can be a result of a depression in a treated solar damaged eye.

The duration of exposure necessary to cause injury varies with the intensity of light, and also affects the possibility and length of recovery.

9. TFTTF

Hypotony may be defined both statistically and clinically. The statistical definition of hypotony is intraocular pressure (IOP) less than 6.5 mmHg, which is more than 3 standard deviations below the mean IOP. The clinical definition of hypotony is IOP low enough to result in vision loss. The vision loss from low IOP may be caused by corneal edema, astigmatism, cystoid macular edema, or maculopathy. Hypotonic maculopathy is characterised by a low IOP associated with fundus abnormalities, including chorioretinal folds, optic nerve head oedema in the acute setting, and vascular tortuosity.

Hypotonic maculopathy may occur after ocular inflammation, trauma, or surgery. Most cases are secondary to glaucoma filtration surgery with a reported incidence of 1.3–18%. Furthermore, the risk of hypotonic maculopathy increases with the use of antifibrosis agents during glaucoma surgery.

Some causes of unilateral hypotony:

- Mitomycin C (MMC) toxicity of the ciliary body
- Overfiltration
- Bleb/wound Leak
- Iridocyclitis
- Cyclodialysis
- Ciliochoroidal Detachment
- Retinal Detachment
- Scleral perforation.

Some causes of bilateral hypotony:

- Osmotic Dehydration
- Diabetic coma
- Uremia
- Myotonic Dystrophy.

The anteroposterior diameter of the eye shortens which can manifest as a refractive hyperopic shift. Anterior bowing of the lamina cribrosa in the optic nerve leads to restricted axoplasmic flow causing disc swelling in the acute phase. Patients with advanced optic nerve disease may not develop optic nerve head swelling and edema due to fewer viable axons.

10. TTTTT

Degenerative myopia is associated with the following;

- Down syndrome
- Pierre-Robin Syndrome
- Prematurity
- Stickler Syndrome
- Marfan's syndrome
- Ehlers-Danlos syndrome
- Noonan syndrome.

Clinical features of degenerative myopia;

- Pale fundus with visible choroidal vessels
- Chorioretinal atrophy

- Lattice degeneration
- Lacquer cracks
- Fuchs spot
- Staphyloma
- Tilted disc.

11. FTTFT

Tay-Sachs disease is a genetic disorder inherited in an autosomal recessive fashion. It affects the retina, the brain and spinal cord. It usually presents in the first few months of life with the inability to turn over, sit or crawl. The patients usually die in the first 3–4 years of life.

Tay-Sachs and the retina; Since the alpha subunit of the enzyme Beta-hexosaminidase A is defective there is accumulation of ganglioside GM2 in the retinal neurones leading to toxicity. It forms a white tinge around the macula where retinal ganglion cells are the thickest. The central macula is relatively free from neurones so ganglioside GM2 does not accumulate leaving the perifoveal area bright red—the 'cherry-red spot'. It is associated with hearing loss.

Tay–Sachs disease is caused by a genetic mutation in the HEXA gene on chromosome 15.

References

1. Martin D, Maguire M, Fine S, Ying G, Jaffe G, Grunwald J et al. Comparison of Age-related Macular Degeneration Treatments Trials (CATT) Research Group, 3rd. Ranibizumab and bevacizumab for treatment of neovascular age-related macular degeneration: two-year results. Ophthalmology. 2012;119(7):1388–98.
2. Bevacizumab. The American Society of Health-System Pharmacists. Archived from the original on 20 December 2016. Retrieved 8 December 2016.
3. Garg SP, Dada T, Talwar D, Biswas NR. Endogenous cortisol profile in patients with central serous chorioretinopathy. Br J Ophthalmol. 1997;81(11):962–4. https://doi.org/10.1136/bjo.81.11.962. PMC 1722041. PMID 9505819.
4. Lee JY. Spironolactone in the treatment of non-resolving central serous chorioretinopathy: a comparative analysis. Acta Ophthalmologica. 2016;94. https://doi.org/10.1111/j.1755-3768.2016.0285.
5. Singh RP, Sears JE, Bedi R, Schachat AP, Ehlers JP, Kaiser PK. Oral eplerenone for the management of chronic central serous chorioretinopathy. Int J Ophthalmol. 2015;8(2): 310–4. https://doi.org/10.3980/j.issn.2222-3959.2015.02.17. PMC 4413566. PMID 25938046.
6. Pecora JL. Ibuprofen in the treatment of central serous chorioretinopathy. Ann Ophthalmol. 1978;10(11):1481–3. PMID 727624.
7. What Causes Macular Edema. American Academy of Ophthalmology.
8. https://emedicine.medscape.com/article/1190444-overview.
9. Gass JD. Hypotony maculopathy. In: Bellows JG, editor. Contemporary ophthalmology. Honouring Sir Stewart Duke-Elder. Baltimore: Williams & Wilkins; 1972. p. 343–66.
10. Costa VP, Arceiri ES. Hypotony maculopathy. Acta Ophthalmol. 2007:586–97.
11. Tay Sachs Disease. NORD (National Organization for Rare Disorders). 2017. Marinetti, GV. Disorders of lipid metabolism. Springer Science & Business Media; 2012. p. 205. ISBN 9781461595649. Archived from the original on 2017-11-05.

Chapter 6
Vitreous and Vitreoretinal Interface Pathology

1. Posterior vitreous detachment (PVD) [1, 2];

    (a) commoner in simple myopia
    (b) syneresis refers to vitreous condensation
    (c) mostly spontaneous
    (d) can be caused by panretinal photocoagulation (PRP)
    (e) can be caused by uveitis.

2. Shafer sign [3–5];

    (a) also know as 'tobacco dust'
    (b) caused by dispersed red blood cells in the vitreous
    (c) caused by condensed hyalocytes
    (d) is not a sensitive sign of retinal pathology
    (e) should be ignored in the absence of retinal symptoms.

3. Epiretinal Membrane (ERM) symptoms include [6];

    (a) micropsia
    (b) macropsia
    (c) aniseikonia
    (d) diplopia
    (e) myodesopsia.

4. Surgical treatment of ERM;

    (a) the earlier the surgery, the better
    (b) post-op there is a 2-line improvement in VA in <50% of cases
    (c) 25G pars plana vitrectomy is the best surgical option
    (d) membrane peel is low risk surgery
    (e) visual acuity improvement is instant in most of the cases.

© Springer Nature Switzerland AG 2020
M. J. Gouder, *The Retina*, https://doi.org/10.1007/978-3-030-48591-7_6

5. Asteroid Hyalosis [7];

    (a) common in the young
    (b) are mobile deposits
    (c) commonly found in the diabetic eye
    (d) cause severe visual impairment
    (e) highly refractile.

6. Causes of cellophane maculopathy [8];

    (a) chorioretinitis
    (b) panretinal photocoagulation (PRP)
    (c) thyroid eye disease
    (d) retinal detachment surgery
    (e) trabeculectomy surgery.

7. Causes of Macular holes [9];

    (a) oculocutaneous albinism
    (b) blunt trauma to the eye
    (c) background diabetic retinopathy
    (d) myopia
    (e) epiretinal membranes.

8. Vitreomacular adhesion (VMA) [10];

    (a) there are obvious foveal changes
    (b) always symptomatic
    (c) can lead to vitreomacular traction
    (d) treatment with pars plans vitrectomy
    (e) caused by pseudocyst.

9. Treatment of Full Thickness Macular hole (FTMH) [11, 12];

    (a) 20G pars plana vitrectomy is the standard current treatment
    (b) all the vitreous is removed
    (c) the eye is filled with air at the end of the procedure
    (d) endolaser to secure the hole
    (e) the smaller the macular hole the higher the success rate.

10. Ocriplasmin [11];

    (a) a protease
    (b) dissolves fibronectin and laminin
    (c) successful in 80% of cases
    (d) used in the treatment of CSR
    (e) promotes posterior vitreous detachment.

1 Answers

1. TFTTT
2. TFFFF
3. FTTTF
4. FFTFF
5. FFFFT
6. TTFTF
7. FTFTF
8. FFTFF
9. FFFFT
10. TTFFT.

2 Answers in Detail

1. TFTTT

A posterior vitreous detachment (PVD) is defined as the separation of the posterior hyaloid face/membrane (PHM) from the neurosensory retina anywhere posterior to the vitreous base. The vitreous base does not detaches itself. At birth, the vitreous fills the back of the eye and normally has Jello-like consistency. As one ages, the vitreous undergoes "syneresis," in which it becomes more fluid or liquid-like. The pockets of fluid in the vitreous cavity give the patient a sensation of "floaters" or "cobwebs." As the pockets of fluid collapse on themselves, they gently pull on the retina giving the patient a sensation of "flashes of light" or photopsias. Eventually, the vitreous may completely separate from the neurosensory retina, which is called a posterior vitreous detachment or "PVD" that is confirmed clinically with observation of Weiss ring on funduscopic examination. This usually occurs in one eye at a time, but a PVD in the contralateral eye often occur 6–24 months later. In high myopia, PVD develops increasingly with age and the degree of myopia. As the vitreous gel separates, it may cause a tear in the neurosensory retina which is fragile and thin like a piece of tissue paper. A retinal tear can allow the liquid part of the vitreous to escape behind the retina and separate the retina from its underlying attachments. This is known as a rhegmatogenous retinal detachment. Typically, however, the vitreous separates without any ill effects on the retina.

2. TFFFF

Shafer sign is also known as 'tobacco dust' and represent pigment granules in the anterior vitreous as visible on slit lamp examination with the beam focussed on the retrolental space. They are also mobile and originate from the RPE. Hence their presence is very indicative of a retinal break where RPE cells can escape through the damaged neurosensory retina to reach the vitreous.

These pigments are larger and darker than red blood cells. Red blood cells can also be seen in the retrolental space in a case of haemorrhagic PVD.

Hyalocytes occur in the peripheral part of the vitreous body, and may produce hyaluronic acid, collagen, fibrils, and hyaluronan. Hyalocytes are star-shaped (stellate) cells with oval nuclei.

In a study involving 200 eyes presenting with an acute PVD, 25 were found to have an associated retinal break, 23 of which were also Shafer sign positive. In 115 eyes presenting for retinal detachment repair, 111 had an associated PVD and were found to be Shafer sign positive. Symptomatology was not predictive of an associated retinal break in the PVD group or in those presenting with a retinal detachment.

The increased use of Shafer's sign is recommended as a valuable aid in determining which patients require urgent referral for an expert retinal examination. It is not possible to predict those patients with a retinal break secondary to PVD on the basis of symptomatology alone.

3. FTTTF

Epiretinal membrane (also called macular pucker) is a disease of the eye in response to changes in the vitreous humor or more rarely, diabetes. Sometimes, as a result of immune system response to protect the retina, cells converge in the macular area as the vitreous ages and pull away in posterior vitreous detachment (PVD). PVD can create minor damage to the retina, stimulating exudate, inflammation, and leucocyte response. These cells can form a transparent fibrocellular layer gradually and, like all scar tissue, tighten to create tension on the retina which may bulge and pucker, or even cause swelling or macular edema. Often this results in distortions of vision that are clearly visible as bowing when looking at lines on chart paper (or an Amsler grid) within the macular area, or central 1.0 degree of visual arc. Usually it occurs in one eye first, and may cause binocular diplopia or double vision if the image from one eye is too different from the image of the other eye. The distortions can make objects look different in size (usually larger = macropsia), especially in the central portion of the visual field, creating a localised or field dependent aniseikonia that cannot be fully corrected optically with glasses. Myodesopsia is the perception of floaters and is more associated with posterior vitreous detachment rather than ERM.

4. FFTFF

Surgery is not usually recommended unless the distortions are severe enough to interfere with daily living, since there are the usual hazards of pars plana vitrectomy (PPV) surgery which include endophthalmitis and a possibility of retinal detachment. Recurrence of the disease is very rare and combined ERM-ILM peel has been advocated for better outcomes but remains debatable. 25G- or even 27G PPV with or without cataract extraction is the preferred treatment. The vitreous is replaced with balanced salt solution (BSS) and no gas tamponade is indicated. In macular pucker ie when the fibrocellular epiretinal membrane contracts and distorts the normal architecture of the fovea, macular and paramacular area, the visual acuity improvement is more prominent but sometimes visual improvement does not occur for several months postoperatively.

5. FFFFT

See Table 6.1.

6. TTFTF

The scar tissue is stimulated to grow by injury to the eye. The most common type of "injury" is the separation of the jelly (vitreous) in the centre of the eye from the retina, which occurs in most people during the ageing process. The vitreous is made of water and a network of tiny fibres. When these fibres separate from the retina, they tug on it and this can cause enough damage to stimulate growth of scar tissue. Alternatively, the scar tissue growth may be stimulated by inflammation in the eye, trauma, and perhaps, rarely, cataract surgery.

Thyroid eye disease and the hypotony which can follow trabeculectomy surgery causes choroidal folds and not cellophane maculopathy.

7. FTFTF

Enough mechanical force can be transmitted to the posterior segment in a blunt trauma setting if the object hits the eye directly. This alters the attachments of the vitreous in the area around the fovea leading to distorted anatomy and macular hole formation. Usually in the early stages, the diagnosis is difficult and only clinically evident on OCT. Advanced proliferative diabetic retinopathy can lead to formation of macular hole if there are sufficient tangential tractional forces around the fovea. Myopia is also a cause especially in pathological progressive myopia. The thin retina is a risk factor and anomalous vitreous attachments. Epiretinal membranes cause pseudoholes and not actual macular holes.

Table 6.1 Comparison between asteroid hyalosis and synchysis scintillans

Feature	Asteroid hyalosis	Synchysis scintillans
Age	Senile	Young/pre-senile
Incidence	Rare	Extremely rare
Laterality	Usu. unilateral	Usu. bilateral
Chemistry	Calcium soap, hydroxylapatite, calcium-laden lipids attached to the hyaluronic acid framework of vitreous	Cholesterol crystals
Appearance	Spherical, white-yellow, refractile	Highly-refractive, multicoloured, flat, angular or disc-shaped
Co-morbid findings	Rare, if any usu. DM, hypercholesterolaemia	Secondary to other ocular pathologies such as tumours
Vitreous state	Normal	Syneretic
Visual acuity	Normal	Variable depending on the co-morbid state of the eye

8. FFTFF

In vitreomacular adhesion (VMA) there is partial vitreous detachment around the perifoveal area but the posterior vitreous face is still attached above the fovea itself but does not distort any anatomy of it since there is no traction yet. Hence this is asymptomatic. In vitreomacular traction (VMT) eventual traction development can lead to local distortion of the foveal contour and intraretinal morphological changes around the fovea such as elevation of the fovea itself from the RPE.

9. FFFFT

Full thickness macular holes are treated with 25G or 27G pars plana vitrectomy with fluid-air exchange and insertion of gas tamponade—usually sulfurhexafluoride (SF6) or perfluoropropane (C3F8). When these two gases are compared the macular hole closure rate was similar with sulfurhexafluoride and perfluoropropane, irrespective of hole size, stage, or duration. However, sulfurhexafluoride exhibited a decreased incidence of cataract and ocular hypertension with shorter tamponade duration. Perfluoropropane may have a role as the preferred endotamponading agent in failed primary surgeries. The use of air as endotamponade is not indicated as it is replaced after a couple of days with aqueous produced by the ciliary body. Core vitrectomy is done. In FTMH there is usually already a PVD and all the vitreous above the macula is removed. Some peripheral vitreous is removed making sure the crystalline lens is not touched by the cutter or light-pipe. Any pre-existing cataracts are usually removed as the gas itself will enhance nuclear sclerosis in the post-op period. Endolaser is never used around the macula. Preoperative VA, mid-hole diameter, and base-hole diameter are correlated with anatomic success in macular hole surgery. An excellent surgical prognosis exists for macular holes with mid-hole diameter less than 500 microns and base-hole less than 1000 microns. Macular holes are more common in older females.

10. TTFFT

Ocriplasmin is a recombinant protease with activity against fibronectin and laminin, components of the vitreoretinal interface. It is used for treatment of symptomatic vitreomacular adhesion, for which it received FDA approval in 2012. It works by dissolving the proteins (laminin and fibronectin) that link the vitreous to the macula, resulting in posterior detachment of the vitreous from the retina. Laminin and fibronectin are actively involved in vitreoretinal attachment. Ocriplasmin induces posterior vitreous detachment. Phase III clinical trials demonstrated that a single intravitreal treatment with Ocriplasmin induced a 26.5% of posterior vitreous detachment compared to 10.5 in placebo controls.

References

1. Gauger E, Chin EK, Sohn EH. Vitreous syneresis: an impending Posterior Vitreous Detachment (PVD). University of Iowa Health Care: Ophthalmology and Visual Sciences; See "Discussion" following "Clinical Course". 17 November 2014.
2. Yonemoto J, Noda Y, Masuhara N, Ohno S. Age of onset of posterior vitreous detachment. Curr Opin Ophthalmol. 1996;7(3):73–6. https://doi.org/10.1097/00055735-199606000-00012 PMID 10163464.
3. Tanner V, Harle D, Tan J, Foote B, Williamson TH, Chignell AH. Acute posterior vitreous detachment: the predictive value of vitreous pigment and symptomatology. Br J Ophthalmol. 2000;84(11):1264–8.
4. Sommer F, Brandl F, Weiser B, Tesmar J, Blunk T, Göpferich A. FACS as useful tool to study distinct hyalocyte populations. Exp Eye Res. 2009;88(5):995–9. https://doi.org/10.1016/j.exer.2008.11.026 PMID 19073178.
5. Paulsen DF. Chapter 24. Sense organs. In: Histology and cell biology: examination and board review. 5th ed. Stamford, Conn.: Appleton & Lange; 2010. ISBN 978-0071476652.
6. de Wit GC. Retinally-induced aniseikonia. Binocul Vis Strabismus Q;22(2):96–101. PMID 17688418.
7. http://visionmagazineonline.co.za/2018/04/01/asteroid-hyalosis-versus-synchysis-scintillans/.
8. https://www.brightfocus.org/macular/article/macular-pucker.
9. Salter AB1, Folgar FA, Weissbrot J, Wald KJ. Macular hole surgery prognostic success rates based on macular hole size. Ophthalmic Surg Lasers Imaging. 2012;43(3):184–9. https://doi.org/10.3928/15428877-20120102-05. Epub 2012 Feb 9.
10. Yoanmb—Own work, CC BY-SA 4.0, https://commons.wikimedia.org/w/index.php?curid=62739301.
11. Stalmans, P; Benz, MS; Gandorfer, A; Kampik, A; Girach, A; Pakola, S; Haller, JA; MIVI-TRUST Study, Group (Aug 16. Enzymatic vitreolysis with ocriplasmin for vitreomacular traction and macular holes. New Eng J Med. 2012;367(7):606–15.
12. Modi A, Giridhar A, Gopalakrishnan M. Sulfurhexafluoride (SF6) versus perfluoropropane (C3F8) gas as tamponade in macular hole surgery. Retina. 2017;37(2):283–90. https://doi.org/10.1097/iae.0000000000001124.

Chapter 7
Drug-Induced Retinopathies

1. Tamoxifen [1, 2];

    (a) is an anti-progesterone
    (b) used in treatment of certain brain tumours
    (c) can cause a crystalline maculopathy
    (d) the maculopathy is reversible
    (e) causes cystoid macular oedema.

2. Chloroquine [3, 4];

    (a) hydroxychloroquine (HCQ) is safer than chloroquine
    (b) used in the treatment of autoimmune disease
    (c) cumulative effect on the retina
    (d) retina screening is essential
    (e) can produce a peripheral visual defect.

3. Bull's eye maculopathy is seen in [5];

    (a) chloroquine toxicity
    (b) Stickler's syndrome
    (c) ARMD
    (d) trauma
    (e) Bardet-Biedl syndrome.

4. Chloroquine/hydroxychloroquine toxicity;

    (a) Asians less prone to develop retinopathy
    (b) used regularly in SLE
    (c) is very rare
    (d) is completely reversible
    (e) binds to pigmented ocular tissues.

© Springer Nature Switzerland AG 2020
M. J. Gouder, *The Retina*, https://doi.org/10.1007/978-3-030-48591-7_7

5. Sildenafil [6, 7];

    (a) is a selective inhibitor of phosphodiesterase type 5 (PDE5)
    (b) can cause retinal arteriole dilation
    (c) causes transient blue/green tinge to vision
    (d) treatment for pulmonary arterial hypertension
    (e) do not cross the blood-retina barrier.

6. Phenothiazines [8];

    (a) include chlorpromazine and thioridazine
    (b) thioridazine is more toxic to the retina than chlorpromazine
    (c) cause a salt and pepper retinopathy
    (d) causes a non-pigmentary type of retinopathy
    (e) can also affect the lids.

7. Drug-induced crystalline maculopathy is associated with [7–10];

    a) tamoxifen
    b) canthaxanthine
    c) methoxyflurane
    d) nitrofurantoin
    e) ethambutol.

8. Desferrioxamine-related ocular toxicity [11];

    (a) includes night blindness and peripheral visual field defects
    (b) does not affect colour vision
    (c) ERG is unchanged
    (d) expect pigmentary mottling of the retina
    (e) RAPD.

9. Talc retinopathy [12];

    (a) common in long term iv drug abusers
    (b) can cause a crystalline retinopathy
    (c) can cause branch retinal artery emboli
    (d) associated with a patent foramen ovale
    (e) always symptomatic.

10. Drug-induced retinopathies;

    (a) clofazimine causes Bull's eye maculopathy
    (b) desferrioxamine can cause a vitelliform retinal pigment epithelial changes
    (c) MEK inhibitors can cause CSR
    (d) corticosteroids can cause CSR
    (e) alkyl nitrites can cause a toxic maculopathy.

1 Answers

1. FTTTT
2. TTTTF
3. TFTTT
4. FTFFT
5. TTTTF
6. TTTFT
7. TTTTF
8. TFFTT
9. TTTTF
10. TTTTT.

2 Answers in Detail

1. FTTTT

Tamoxifen citrate, an oral anti-oestrogen, is most commonly used in low dosages (20 mg/d) as an adjuvant therapy for breast cancer. At significantly higher dosages (200 mg/d), it has also been used to treat malignant astrocytoma of the brain. Of its well-documented ocular toxic effects, potentially the most devastating is the development of crystalline maculopathy with associated cystoid macular edema (CMO).

Clinically it causes extensive, usually bilateral, refractile, white perifoveal crystalline deposits. These deposits can extend up to the periphery in the retina. Treatment consists of cessation of the medication, which may stabilise vision but rarely results in its recovery. It can be treated with repeated intravitreal bevacizumab (1.25 mg standard dose). Toxic effects appear to be dose related, with cumulative doses exceeding 100 g predisposing to vortex keratopathy, lens opacities, optic neuritis, retinal pigment epithelium abnormalities, crystalline maculopathy, and CME but these findings are rare in those receiving lower-dose therapy for breast cancer. High-resolution OCT can show tamoxifen-associated CME in the absence of crystals. The crystalline retinal deposits are classically confined to the nerve fibre and inner plexiform layers and are hypothesised to represent areas of axonal degeneration.

2. TTTTF

Chloroquine has been replaced by the much safer hydroxychloroquine. This medication is used in the prevention and treatment of certain types of malaria. It is also used in the treatment of rheumatic arthritis and some dermatological conditions such as discoid lupus, lichen planus and porphyria cutanea tarda. It is an emerging treatment option in oncology such as non-small cell lung tumours and paediatric inflammatory disorders such as interstitial lung disease in children. Hydroxychloroquine binds to the melanin in the RPE causing dysfunction. Hence the total ingestion must always be calculated. It usually produces a paracentral scotoma, a central scotoma with reading difficulty. The peripheral visual field can be affected in advanced stages only. Initially the colour vision is unaffected but can deteriorate in advanced stages.

Chloroquine was developed in 1939, and through additional of an hydroxyl group, its analogue, hydroxychloroquine was developed soon after and has been used since the 1960s.

3. TFTTT

Causes of Bull's Eye maculopathy;

- Chloroquine/Hydroxychloroquine
- Stargardt's disease
- ARMD
- Clofazimine—used in the treatment of leprosy
- Cone dystrophy
- Cone-Rod dystrophy
- Leber congenital amaurosis
- Sorsby central areolar choroidal dystrophy
- Trauma.

4. FTFFT

Hydroxychloroquine retinal toxicity is far more common than previously considered; an overall prevalence of 7.5% was identified in patients taking the drug for more than 5 years, rising to almost 20% after 20 years of treatment. It causes irreversible visual loss due to retinal toxicity. Asian patients with hydroxychloroquine retinopathy may demonstrate an extra-macular or pericentral pattern of disease so visual field testing and retinal imaging should include a wider field for screening in this group.

There is widespread binding of chloroquine in pigmented ocular tissues: the RPE, iris, choroid and ciliary body with eventual accumulation observed in the retina.

5. TTTTF

Sildenafil is a medication used to treat erectile dysfunction and pulmonary arterial hypertension. Onset is typically within 20 minutes and lasts for about 2 hours. Sildenafil is a selective cGMP-specific phosphodiesterase type 5 inhibitor which causes retinal arteriole and venue dilation. It exerts a minor inhibitory action against PDE6, which is present exclusively in rod and cone photoreceptors. This class of vasodilators is capable of crossing the blood-retina barrier.

Ocular effects;

- blurred vision
- Cyanopsia (blue/green tinge to vision)
- non-arteritic ischaemic optic neuropathy (NAION).

6. TTTFT

Phenothiazines are used in the treatment of psychoses. These include chlorprom-azine and thioridazine, the latter being more toxic to the retina than the former. Initially RPE stippling occurs in the posterior pole followed by a nummular (plaque-like) RPE atrophy which leads to a more widespread atrophic and pig-mentary retinopathy which is similar to choroideremia. Thioridazine is also asso-ciated with dark adaption issues.

7. TTTTF

Tamoxifen is described in detail above. Canthaxanthin is a keto-carotenoid pig-ment widely distributed in nature. A reversible deposition of canthaxanthin crys-tals was discovered in the retina of a limited number of people who had consumed very high amounts of canthaxanthin via sun-tanning pills but after stopping the pills, the deposits disappeared. However, the level of canthaxanthin intake in the affected individuals was many times greater than that which could ever be con-sumed via poultry products (canthaxanthin is added as a supplement in many ani-mal feeds including poultry).

Methoxyflurane is a fluorinated hydrocarbon anaesthetic used in pain manage-ment in trauma cases.

8. TFFTT

Desferrioxamine can be associated with;

– rapidly deteriorating symptoms of night blindness and peripheral visual field loss (annular scotomas) and impaired colour vision
– vitelliform kind of maculopathy
– pigmentary retinopathy and optic neuropathy (expect RAPD).

IVFA shows speckled hyper-fluorescence with well-demarcated areas of blocked fluorescence.

9. TTTTF

Talc retinopathy is a recognised ocular condition characterised by the presence of small, yellow, glistening crystals found inside small retinal vessels and within dif-ferent retinal layers. The crystals are thought to be secondary to emboli derived from talc which is an insoluble inert particulate filler material (excipient) used in preparation of certain oral (methylphenidate hydrochloride, methadone, pentazo-cine and amphetamine), inhalational (crack cocaine), and intravenous (cocaine and heroin) drugs. When these oral tablets are crushed and injected intravenously, most of the talc particles get trapped in the pulmonary vasculature except for very small particles (<7 μm) that escape from the pulmonary capillary bed and reach the eye through systemic circulation. Ocular findings usually develop after chronic intravenous drug abuse and range from asymptomatic crystalline retinopathy to ischaemic manifestations of capillary non perfusion and neovascularization.

10. TTTTT

Clofazimine is a phenazine dye and believed to work by interfering with DNA. It is a medication used together with rifampicin and dapsone to treat leprosy. It is specifically used for multibacillary leprosy and erythema nodosum leprosum. It can cause Bull's eye maculopathy.

A MEK inhibitor is a chemical or drug that inhibits the mitogen-activated protein kinase enzymes MEK1 and/or MEK2. They can be used to affect the MAPK/ERK pathway which is often overactive in some cancers. Hence MEK inhibitors have potential for treatment of some cancers, especially BRAF-mutated melanoma, and KRAS/BRAF mutated colorectal cancer. It can cause a multifocal serous retinal detachments.

Alkyl nitrites "poppers" are recreational drugs. It is inhaled to induce euphoria and relax smooth muscles. They can cause toxic maculopathy. Usually young, the patient presents with a central scotoma. Typically there is a yellow spot on the fovea.

References

1. Rahimy E, Sarraf D. Bevacizumab therapy for tamoxifen-induced crystalline retinopathy and severe cystoid macular edema. Arch Ophthalmol. 2012;130(7):931–2. https://doi.org/10.1001/archophthalmol.2011.2741.
2. Yusuf IH, Sharma S, Luqmani R, Downes SM. Hydroxychloroquine retinopathy. Eye (Lond). 2017;31(6):828–45. Published online 2017 Mar 10. https://doi.org/10.1038/eye.2016.298.
3. Gass JDM. Stereoscopic atlas of macular diseases: diagnosis and treatment, vol. 1. 4th ed. St. Louis: Mo Mosby–Year Book Inc; 1997. p. 1–9.
4. Yam JC, Kwok AK. Ocular toxicity of hydroxychloroquine. Hong Kong Med J. 2006;12(4):294–304.
5. Nasser F, Kurtenbach A, Kohl S, Obermaier C, Stingl K, Zrenner E. Retinal dystrophies with bull's-eye maculopathy along with negative ERGs. Doc Ophthalmol. 2019;139(1):45–57. Epub 2019 Apr 3. https://doi.org/10.1007/s10633-019-09694-7.
6. Pache M, Meyer P, Prünte C, et al. Sildenafil induces retinal vasodilatation in healthy subjects. Brit J Ophthalmol. 2002;86:156–8.
7. Laties A, Zrenner E. Viagra (sildenafil citrate) and ophthalmology. Prog Retin Eye Res. 2002;21(5):485–506.
8. Richa S, Yazbek J. Ocular adverse effects of common psychotropic agents: a review. CCNS Drugs. 2010;24(6):501–26. https://doi.org/10.2165/11533180-000000000-00000.
9. Hueber A, Rosentreter A, Severin M. Canthaxanthin retinopathy: long-term observations. Ophthalmic Res. 2011;46(2):103–6. https://doi.org/10.1159/000323813.
10. Porter KM, Dayan AD, Dickerson S, Middleton PM. The role of inhaled methoxyflurane in acute pain management. Open Access Emerg Med. 2018;10:149–164. https://doi.org/10.2147/OAEM.S181222
11. Simon S, Athanasiov PA, Jain R, Raymond G, Gilhotra JS. Desferrioxamine-related ocular toxicity: a case report. Indian J Ophthalmol. 2012;60(4):315–17. https://doi.org/10.4103/0301-4738.98714.
12. Soliman MK, Sarwar S, Hanout M, Sadiq MA, Agarwal A, Gulati V, Nguyen QD, Sepah YJ. High-resolution adaptive optics findings in talc retinopathy. Int J Retina Vitreous. 2015;1:10. Published online 2015 Jul 24. https://doi.org/10.1186/s40942-015-0009-4.

Chapter 8
Vitreoretinal Surgery

1. Common indications for vitrectomy include [1]:

   (a) proliferative vitreoretinopathy (PVR)
   (b) persistent vitreous haemorrhage
   (c) pre-proliferative diabetic retinopathy
   (d) retinopathy of prematurity (ROP)
   (e) vitreous biopsy.

2. Advantages of using smaller gauge trocars in PPV include [2]:

   (a) shorter theatre time
   (b) sutures are never used
   (c) quicker post-operative recovery and patient comfort
   (d) can be used in paediatric cases
   (e) less corneal astigmatism.

3. Disadvantages of small gauge vitrectomy [3]:

   (a) higher infusion and aspiration pressures needed
   (b) greater instrument flexion
   (c) ideal for complex vitreoretinal diseases
   (d) increased risk of intra-operative cannula dislocation
   (e) early postoperative hypotony.

4. Features of the cannula system in pars plana vitrectomy [4–6]:

   (a) the 'gauge' relates to the internal diameter of vitrectomy instruments
   (b) the higher the gauge number, the larger the diameter of the instruments
   (c) the cannula system creates less traction on the vitreous base
   (d) lessens trauma to the wound border
   (e) cannulas maintain the alignment between the conjunctiva and sclera.

© Springer Nature Switzerland AG 2020
M. J. Gouder, *The Retina*, https://doi.org/10.1007/978-3-030-48591-7_8

5. Postoperative hypotony in PPV can be associated with [7]:

   (a) choroidal detachment
   (b) choroidal haemorrhage
   (c) hypotonic maculopathy
   (d) inadequate endotamponade
   (e) higher rates of endophthalmitis.

6. Complications of intraocular gas in vitreoretinal surgery include [8]:

   (a) posterior polar cataract
   (b) glaucoma
   (c) central retinal artery occlusion
   (d) macular burns after laser
   (e) endophthalmitis.

7. Complications of silicone oil [9]:

   (a) posterior polar cataract
   (b) open-angle glaucoma
   (c) band keratopathy
   (d) retinal toxicity
   (e) subconjunctival oil is easy to remove.

8. Refractive changes in a patient with Silicone oil:

   (a) hypermetropic shift in phakic patients
   (b) hypermetropic shift in aphakic patients
   (c) hypermetropic shift in pseudophakic patients
   (d) hypermetropic shift in myopes
   (e) silicon oil has the same refractive index as vitreous.

9. Retinal detachment pathophysiology:

   (a) all retinal layers detach
   (b) the vitreous base commonly detaches in peripheral retinal detachment
   (c) atrophic retinal holes are caused due to degeneration
   (d) atrophic retinal holes are common in the periphery
   (e) retinal dialysis is associated with trauma.

1   Answers

1. TTFTT
2. TFTTT
3. TTFTT

4. FFTTT
5. TTTTT
6. FTTTT
7. FTTTF
8. TFTTF
9. FFTFT.

2 Answers in Detail

1. TTFTT

Indications of vitreoretinal surgery;

- dislocated lens fragments during complicated cataract surgery with posterior capsule tear
- dislocated intraocular implants during or after cataract surgery
- recurrent vitreous haemorrhage not resolving on its own
- proliferative diabetic retinopathy with or without tractional retinal detachment
- rhegmatogenous retinal detachment
- symptomatic epiretinal membranes and macular pucker
- macular holes
- non-resolving symptomatic vitreomacular traction syndrome
- severe endophthalmitis
- trauma with perforation and presence of intraocular foreign body
- retinopathy of prematurity (using special smaller gauge trocars)
- subretinal haemorrhage
- choroidal neovascular membrane (indication falling out of fashion)
- diagnostic vitrectomy to obtain vitreous biopsy or to biopsy a lesion.

In background or preproliferative diabetic retinopathy vitrectomy is not indicated and other non-invasive techniques are used like argon laser and/or intravitreal anti-VEGFs injections and intravitreal steroid (short and longer-acting).

2. TFTTT

Currently 23G and 25G vitrectomy is the most popular. 27G is indicated for quick vitrectomies such as floaterectomy.

The smaller the gauge the less the trauma to surrounding tissues but instruments tend to become less stiffer and tend to bend easily limiting the manipulation inside the eye.

Advantages of small gauge vitrectomy:

- less surgical trauma to the pars plana
- self-sealing wounds and hence most of the time it is sutureless surgery but this is not always. If the wound leaks one needs to suture the wound with 6/0 or 7/0 vicryl preferably undyed

- less operating time hence more time for other surgery
- less manipulation of the pars plana hence less astigmatism
- faster recovery
- less conjunctival scarring
- ideal in paediatric cases where pars plana is narrow.

3. TTFTT

Small gauge vitrectomy utilising 23- and 25-gauge instrumentation has definite advantages, but also limitations, due to the physics of smaller instruments and sutureless surgery. Higher infusion and aspiration pressures are needed to remove the vitreous using 23- and 25-gauge probes.

The advantages have been outlined above. A disadvantage is greater instrument flexion than 20-gauge probes, making small gauge vitrectomy more appropriate for indications such as vitreous opacities, epiretinal membranes, macular holes, and simple retinal detachments.

Small gauge vitrectomy is not indicated for complex vitreoretinal disease where extensive prolonged segmentation of fibrovascular membranes is required. Hence cases involving prolonged work such as in proliferative diabetic retinopathy or proliferative vitreoretinopathy should be done with larger gauge surgery i.e. 23G. There are also some increased complications related to small gauge vitrectomy, including intra-operatively dislocation of cannulas, early postoperative hypotony, choroidal detachment, and possibly an increased risk of infectious endophthalmitis.

4. FFTTT

The gauge relates to the outer diameter of vitrectomy instruments and the higher the number the smaller the diameter of instruments (Table 8.1).

The trocar/cannula system theoretically creates less traction on the vitreous base during instrument entry and exit. A 20G sclerotomy involves a lot of manipulation in the pars plana due to the use of vicryl sutures to secure the wound at the end of procedure. This increases the risk of bleeding and complications compared to the smaller gauge cannulas—23G and 25G. Furthermore in the latter small gauge techniques, the cannula is inserted once and this maintains the alignment between the conjunctiva and sclera. This increases the chance of a self-sealing sclerotomy at the end of the procedure and is associated with less wound inflammation and late-onset scleral atrophy at the original site of the wound.

Table 8.1 Vitrectomy cannula gauge outer diameter

17G	1.42 mm
20G	0.89 mm
23G	0.72 mm
25G	0.55 mm
27G	0.4 mm

A disadvantage of smaller gauge cannulas is that since the cannula's internal diameter is smaller, the radius of curvature of intraocular scissors has to be smaller too, resulting in a blunted curve and shorter blades so rendering them less efficient for membrane cutting and dissection when compared to their 20G counterparts. The cannula sleeve may also slightly affect instrument rotation and flexion during globe manipulation, as well as anterior and peripheral access. Placing the sclerotomies closer to the horizontal meridian reduces the need to rotate instruments significantly for peripheral and superior access and avoids displacement of the infusion as the eye is rotated inferiorly.

5. TTTTT

Sutureless surgery can lead to inadequate wound sealing of the sclerotomies. The hypotony is usually transient, but can sometimes be severe, leading to choroidal detachment or haemorrhage, hypotonic maculopathy, or gas escape leading to inadequate tamponade. Furthermore, initial reports suggested higher rates of endophthalmitis.

Post-operative endophthalmitis in small gauge pars plana vitrectomy can be due to:

- contamination from conjunctival flora
- ingress associated with postoperative hypotony
- vitreous wick effect at unsutured sclerotomies.

Studies have shown that straight sclera incision is a higher risk for endophthalmitis than a bevelled one.

6. FTTTT

The ideal gas for vitreoretinal surgery should be nontoxic, inert, insoluble in the aqueous humor, and have a lower water solubility than nitrogen.

When intraocular gases are used they undergo three phases before resorption: expansion, equilibration, and dissolution.

Expansion: the intraocular gas volume rises as the nitrogen diffusion rate into the bubble is greater than the dissolution of the gas into the surrounding tissue fluid compartment.

Equilibration: the concentration of nitrogen in the bubble is equilibrated with the bloodstream, and a small amount of expandable gas diffuses out of the eye.

Dissolution: the partial pressure of all gases in the bubble equals that in the fluid compartment, the dissolution begins.

If the patient lies supine after insertion of gas, this gas comes in contact with the posterior lens surface inducing a posterior subcapsular (cortical) lenticular opacity typically known as 'gas cataract'. Nuclear sclerosis is also associated with intraocular gas but this usually develops at later stage. A posterior polar cataract is usually congenital and the opacity is concentrated near the apex of the posterior aspect of the lens. This is different from gas cataract. To minimise this complication the patient is instructed to avoid the supine position hence there is less gas-crystalline lens contact.

IOP increase in eyes with intraocular tamponade is a common postoperative complication reported in up to 60% of eyes. The mechanism can be open angle, closed angle, or both. In open-angle mechanism, IOP elevation is due to intraocular gas expansion. Closed-angle cases are less common but are usually a result of anterior displacement of the iris-lens diaphragm and iridocorneal apposition with or without pupillary block. Very high IOP can lead to retinal ischaemia and optic nerve damage.

If laser is applied after surgery and the eye is filled with gas the laser beam can be reflected inside the eye causing macular or foveal burn.

Other potential complications of intraocular gas;

– displacement of intraocular lens implant
– myopic shift whilst gas is in situ (50D myopic shift due to the huge difference between refractive index of the lens and air)
– subconjunctival gas from wound leakage
– anterior chamber gas leak from zonular dehiscence or posterior capsule defects.

7. FTTTF

List of Silicone oil-related complication;

• nuclear sclerotic cataract
• posterior capsule thickening in the pseudophakic patient
• glaucoma due to presence of silicon oil in trabecular meshwork
• band keratopathy
• phthisis bulbi
• retinal toxicity
• angle-closure glaucoma in an silicon oil-filled aphakic eye
• decreased vision due to oil emulsification
• subretinal and subchoroidal oil
• subconjunctival oil due to wound leakage (difficult to remove as small bubbles infiltrates the Tenon's layer and cause inflammation).

8. TFTTF

The refractive shift depends on the patient's lens status. Silicone oil has a higher refractive index than vitreous so this difference induces refractive errors. In the phakic patient the anterior surface of the oil bubble is concave and this induces a hypermetropic shift. This also occurs in the pseudophakic patient but to a lesser extent as the IOL has a flatter posterior surface (less concave). In aphakia the anterior surface of the silicone bubble is convex and this promotes a myopic shift. High myopes who are also phakic notice that their myopia is less severe post-op. Aphakic patients will notice that their pre-op high plus lens is less severe in the post-op period.

9. FFTFT

In retinal detachment only the neurosensory retina detaches from the RPE which is the outermost layer of the retina. The vitreous base which straddles across the pars plana, ora serrata and the very peripheral retina remains attached in cases of retinal detachment. The retina also remains anchored at the optic nerve which is an important sign on B-Scan analysis when there is no fundal view and an RD is suspected such as in dense cataract situations. Low intraocular pressure is also another hint that the retina might be detached. Retinal round holes compared to retinal tears are caused by localised retinal degeneration and is usually related to myopia. Retinal tears are caused by the dynamic vitreous traction in incomplete posterior vitreous detachment. In PVD the vitreous commonly remains attached to the vitreous base anteriorly. Atrophic holes are often equatorial and associated with lattice degeneration. Retinal dialysis, commonly occur in the inferotemporal retina and are associated with severe blunt trauma to the eye. Surgically they do well by a 360 degree encirclement.

References

1. Bopp S, Kellner U. Klin Monbl Augenheilkd [Article in German; Abstract available in German from the publisher]. 2019 Feb 18 [Pars plana vitrectomy]. https://doi.org/10.1055/a-0849-0148.
2. Pollack JS, Sabherwal N. Small gauge vitrectomy: operative techniques. Curr Opin Ophthalmol. 2019;30(3):159–64. https://doi.org/10.1097/icu.0000000000000568.
3. Thompson JT. Advantages and limitations of small gauge vitrectomy. Surv Ophthalmol. 2011;56(2):162–72. https://doi.org/10.1016/j.survophthal.2010.08.003.
4. Nagpal M, Paranjpe G, Jain P, Videkar R. Advances in small-gauge vitrectomy. Taiwan Journal of Ophthalmology. 2012;2(1):6–12. https://doi.org/10.1016/j.tjo.2012.01.001.
5. Sana Idrees, Ajay E. Kuriyan, Stephen G. SchwartzJean-Marie, Parel Harry W. Flynn Jr. Recent Developments in Vitreoretinal Surgery. Curr Concepts Ophthalmol:165–99.
6. Rizzo S, Beltling C, Genovesi-Ebert F, di Bartolo E. Incidence of retinal detachment after small-incision, sutureless pars plana vitrectomy compared with conventional 20-gauge vitrectomy in macular hole and epiretinal membrane surgery. Retina. 2010;30(7):1065–71. https://doi.org/10.1097/IAE.0b013e3181cd48b0.
7. Scott IU, Flynn HW Jr, Dev S, et al. Endophthalmitis after 25-gauge and 20-gauge pars plana vitrectomy: incidence and outcomes. Retina. 2008;28(1):138–42. https://doi.org/10.1097/iae.0b013e31815e9313.
8. Kanclerz Piotr, Grzybowski Andrzej. Complications associated with the use of expandable gases in vitrectomy. J Ophthalmol. 2018;2018:8606494.
9. Herbert EN, Habib M, Steel D, Williamson TH. Central scotoma associated with intraocular silicone oil tamponade develops before oil removal. Graefes Arch Clin Exp Ophthalmol. 2006;244(2):248–52. Epub 2005 Jul 27.

Chapter 9
Choroidal and Retinal Tumours

1. Choroidal naevus [1]:

   (a) commoner in dark-skinned people
   (b) usually grow in adulthood
   (c) it is comprised of spindle-cell melanocytes
   (d) needs regular follow-up
   (e) commonly associated with drusen.

2. Choroidal melanoma risk [1]:

   (a) presence of overlying drusen
   (b) presence of subretinal fluid
   (c) acoustic hollowness on B-Scan
   (d) thickness < 2 mm
   (e) absence of a halo.

3. Investigating choroidal pigmentation [2, 3]:

   (a) OCT is essential
   (b) IVFA is very helpful in distinguishing between benign and malignant lesions
   (c) fundus photography is recommended
   (d) US (B-Scan) is very helpful
   (e) autofluorescence is helpful.

4. Choroidal melanoma [4]:

   (a) commonest primary intraocular malignant tumour
   (b) it is a disease of adulthood
   (c) spread is uncommon
   (d) commonly presents with metastasis
   (e) carries a 50% mortality in 10 years.

5. Pathology of choroidal melanoma [5]:

   (a) commonly composed of spindle cells and epithelioid cells
   (b) spindle cells are associated with a better prognosis
   (c) epithelioid cells associated with a worse prognosis
   (d) likes to erode through Bruch's membrane and RPE
   (e) is more common than ciliary body melanoma.

6. Choroidal melanoma—worse prognosis [6]:

   (a) large tumour
   (b) epithelioid cells
   (c) BAP1 mutations
   (d) anterior location
   (e) extrascleral extension.

7. Choroidal Haemangiomas [6, 7]:

   (a) can be solitary or diffuse
   (b) are benign tumours
   (c) associated with retinal detachment
   (d) show typical B-Scan external reflectivity
   (e) associated with Osler–Weber–Rendu syndrome.

8. Clinical manifestations of Retinoblastoma [8]:

   (a) commonly presents with leucokoria
   (b) hyphaema is a common feature
   (c) can mimic orbital cellulitis
   (d) associated with glaucoma
   (e) exophytic type presents with proptosis.

9. Retinoblastoma [8]:

   (a) incidence of 1:16000 life births
   (b) least common primary intraocular malignancy of childhood
   (c) highest incidence in first few months of life
   (d) commonly diagnosed after 6 years of age
   (e) no racial predilection.

10. Retinoblastoma growth [9]:

   (a) endophytic growth leads to retinal detachment
   (b) exophytic growth typically presents with leucokoria
   (c) commonly grows in both the endophytic and exophytic way
   (d) can grow diffusely inside the retina
   (e) diffuse growth is associated with late diagnosis.

11. Retinoblastoma spread [8, 9]:

   (a) anterior spread to conjunctiva
   (b) posterior spread through optic nerve
   (c) haematogenous spread to bones
   (d) can metastasise to brain
   (e) lymphatic spread is rare.

12. Differential diagnosis of leucokoria:

   (a) persistent hyperplastic primary vitreous
   (b) persistent posterior fetal vasculature
   (c) Coats' disease
   (d) pars planitis
   (e) retinopathy of prematurity.

13. von Hippel-Lindau (VHL) disease is associated with [10]:

   (a) racemose haemangioma
   (b) CNS haemangioma
   (c) pheochromocytoma
   (d) polycythaemia
   (e) renal carcinoma.

14. Congenital hypertrophy of the RPE (CHRPE):

   (a) could be solitary, multifocal and atypical
   (b) solitary CHRPE is commonly found in the peripheral retina
   (c) multifocal CHRPE is always pigmented
   (d) solitary CHRPE is associated with gastrointestinal malignancy
   (e) associated with osteomas of the skull.

15. Cancer-associated retinopathy (CAR) [11, 12]:

   (a) visual symptoms precede the diagnosis of cancer
   (b) typically associated with small-cell bronchial carcinoma
   (c) patients present with a peripheral scotoma
   (d) fundus picture is typically normal
   (e) ERG is normal.

1   Answers

   1. FFTTT
   2. FTTFT
   3. TFTFT
   4. TTFFT

  5. TTTTF
  6. TTTTT
  7. TTTFF
  8. TFTTT
  9. TFTFT
10. FFTTT
11. TTTTF
12. TTTFT
13. FTTTT
14. TTFFT
15. TTFTF.

2 Answers in Detail

1. FFTTT

A choroidal nevus (or benign neoplasm of the choroid) is a greyish-brown pigmented lesion with slightly blurred margins. A choroidal naevus is similar to a large freckle or mole found on the skin. Most choroidal nevi are approximately the same size as the optic disk and are usually round or oval in shape. A choroidal nevus is essentially a benign tumour of the choroid composed of spindle-cell melanocytes which produce melanin.

White people are 500% more likely to have melanoma than African-Americans and three times more likely than Asians to have choroidal nevi.

They typically occur and enlarge during puberty and rarely occur in adulthood. The odds of a choroidal nevus evolving into a melanoma is less than 1%.

2. FTTFT

Risk factors for the growth of choroidal nevus into melanoma:

- thickness > 2 mm
- presence of subretinal fluid
- orange pigment (lipofuscin)
- margin within 3 mm of the optic disc
- ultrasonographic evidence of acoustic hollowness
- absence of halo
- absence of drusen.

Mnemonic:

To Find Small Ocular Melanoma using helpful hints daily

T = Thickness (two)
F = Fluid

S = Symptoms
O = Orange pigment
M = Margin
U, h = US hollowness
H = Halo
D = Drusen.

The presence of three or more risk factors implies more than 50% chance for transformation to melanoma within 5 years.

3. TFTTT

Photographic evidence of any suspicious pigmentation can be captured by using fundus camera. It is useful for monitoring obvious changes such as size and presence of orange pigment and also document how far the lesion is from the optic disc. Optical coherence tomography can quantify the features of the lesion and also detect secondary retinal changes associated with the underlying choroidal lesions. Intravenous fluorescein angiography is not helpful in delineating between benign and malignant lesions. Fundus autofluorescence (FAF) can detect minor orange pigment not clinically obvious on fundus examination or fundus photography. Intense hyperautofluorescence makes the lesion more likely to be a melanoma.

US B-Scan can be used to measure the lesion and acoustic hollowness is a strong indication of malignancy and risk of spread.

FAF is based on the intrinsic property of certain molecules to show transient emission of light, or fluorescence, when illuminated by an external light source. In the eye, many tissues have autofluorescence properties such as the cornea, lens, and the RPE. The main source of FAF is lipofuscin. Lipofuscin accumulates in the RPE from incomplete degradation and digestion of photoreceptor outer segments. Lipofuscin is a mixture of proteins, lipids, and small chromophores. Secondary to decreased or impaired lysosomal activity, the lipofuscin accumulates in the RPE. The intensity of FAF depends mainly on the amount and concentration of lipofuscin. Depending on the intensity of autofluorescence, a lesion may be isoautofluorescent, hypoautofluorescent, or hyperautofluorescent.

4. TTFFT

Choroidal melanoma is the commonest uveal tumour amounting to 80% of such tumours. It is still a very uncommon tumour. These tumours are much more common in adulthood and can metastasise to liver, bone and lung. However it is rare for a tumour to be diagnosed concurrently with metastasis already present. Local Spread is usually through the sclera and vortex veins. It carries a morality of 50% in 10 years.

5. TTFTF

Histologically an ocular melanoma can be composed of spindle cells (Type A and B) or epithelioid cell or a mix of both which is then called mixed type tumour. Spindle cells tumours have cells organised in bundles and carry a better prognosis. Epithelioid cells show a high mitotic rate and hence are more aggressive and commonly metastasise hence associated with a worse prognosis. Metastasis carries a poor prognosis. The tumour likes to assume a collar stud shape when it erodes through Bruch's membrane and then invades the subretinal space. The tumour can be associated with subretinal fluid and retinal detachment (exudative type of retinal detachment).

6. TTTTT

Choroidal melanoma increased mortality:

– the tumour is large (COMS—collaborative ocular melanoma study)
– presence of epithelioid cells (high-mitotic activity)
– anterior location—late diagnosis
– trans-scleral invasion—metastasis
– BAP1 mutations—defect in tumour suppressor gene
– optic nerve extension
– lack of pigmentation.

7. TTTFF

Choroidal haemangiomas are:

– benign vascular hamartomas
– diffuse or solitary
– diffuse associated with Sturge-Weber syndrome
– associated with overlying retinal pigmented epithelium (RPE) changes or orange pigment
– can be associated with associated intraretinal or subretinal fluid
– show high internal reflectivity (A-scan) and acoustic solidity (B-scan). Diffuse hemangioma shows diffuse marked thickening of choroid whereas circumscribed lesions appear as a placoid or oval mass.

8. TFTTT

See Table 9.1.

9. TFTFT

Retinoblastoma has an incidence of 1:16 000 life births and it is the most common primary intraocular malignancy of childhood. Retinoblastoma forms 3% of all childhood malignancies and after uveal melanoma, it is the second most common malignant intraocular tumour. Its highest incidence is in the first few months of life but rarely before 3 months except for in familial cases. It is very rarely diagnosed after 6 years of age and has no racial prediliction.

10. FFTTT

See Fig. 9.1.

Table 9.1 Clinical Manifestations of retinoblastoma; from common to less common features

Feature	Notes
Leucocoria	60%, there is a lack of red reflex in large tumours, retinal detachment, retrolental mass or vitreous opacification due to tumour cells
Strabismus	20%, macular involvement of the tumour can disrupt fusion leading to a squint
Rubeosis iris	17% this occurs in advanced cases due to extensive tumour necrosis releasing angiogenic factors
Red painful eye	Due to inflammation or glaucoma
Poor vision	Due to macular disruption or optic nerve involvement
Asymptomatic	Especially if small and early on the disease
Proptosis	Secondary to optic nerve or orbital extension through scleral emissary veins
Glaucoma	Neovascular or due to angle closure
Orbital cellulitis	As a masquerade syndrome
Unilateral mydriasis	
Heterochromia iridis	
Hyphema	Usually spontaneous, also vitreous haemorrhage
Pseudohypopyon	Seeding of AC in endophytic or diffuse infiltrating tumours

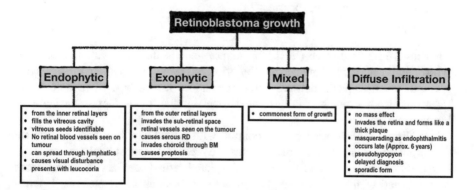

Fig. 9.1 Growth of retinoblastoma

11. TTTTF

See Fig. 9.2.

12. TTTFT

Differential diagnosis of leucocoria;

- retinoblastoma
- persistent hyperplastic primary vitreous (PHPV)
- persistent posterior primary vitreous

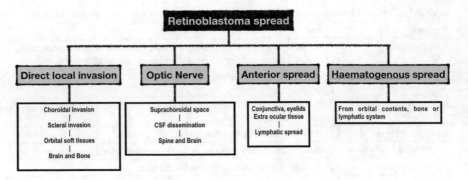

Fig. 9.2 Spread of retinoblastoma

- Coats' disease
- toxocariasis
- familial exudative vitreoretinopathy
- incontinentia pigmenti
- Norrie's disease.

Pars planitis forms the differential diagnosis of vitreous seeds from retinoblastoma but does not usually give leucocoria.

13. FTTTT

Von Hippel-Lindau disease (VHL), is a rare genetic disorder with multisystem involvement [2]. It is characterised by visceral cysts and benign tumors with potential for subsequent malignant transformation. It is a type of phakomatosis that results from a mutation in the Von Hippel-Lindau tumor suppressor gene on chromosome 3p25.3.

Von Hippel-Lindau disease is associated with retinal capillary haemangiomas. If multiple retinal capillary haemangiomas are present it is most likely due to VHL disease. Furthermore 50% of the cases of isolated retinal capillary haemangiomas are associated with VHL disease. The growth of these haemangiomas is dependent on the presence of vascular endothelial growth factor. Usually these retina tumours are detected by screening or present in the clinic with decrease in vision caused my macular exudation or even retinal detachment. So these haemangiomas can leak and even cause haemorrhage leading to tractional retinal detachment if fibrotic bands are formed and pull on the retina.

14. TTFFT

Congenital hypertrophy of the RPE are a group of conditions and could be solitary, multifocal and atypical. Solitary CHRPE is commonly found in the peripheral retina and is a flat, usually round dark grey or black lesion. In the ageing patient there may be loss of pigmentation starting just inside the margin. These solitary CHRPE do not have any association with GI malignancy.

Multifocal CHRPE are usually grouped and form 'bear-tracks' and when they rarely loose pigment can be called 'polar bear tracks'. These lesions, though multifocal, are usually found in one eye compared to the atypical CHRPE which are associated with familial adenomatous polyposis (FAP) which is an autosomal condition associated with polyps throughout the rectum ands colon which can become malignant. Gardner syndrome is characterised by FAP, skull and long bone osteomas, soft tissue tumours and fibromas.

15. TTFTF

Cancer associated retinopathy (CAR) is a member of a spectrum of disease called autoimmune retinopathy. It was first described by Sawyer et al. [11] with three cancer patients presenting with blindness caused by diffuse retinal degeneration. In CAR, retinal degeneration occurs in the presence of auto-antibodies that cross react with tumour-tissue and retinal-tissue antigens which are recognised as foreign. In many instances, visual loss from CAR precedes the diagnosis of cancer. There has been different antibodies isolated against many specific retinal proteins:

- Recoverin
- Carbonic anhydrase II
- Transducin B.

Many different cancers have been associated with CAR. Small cell lung carcinoma, breast cancer, and gynaecologic cancer are the most common cancers associated with CAR. However CAR has been found in other types of lung cancer, colon cancer, mixed Müllerian tumour, skin squamous cancer, kidney cancer, pancreatic, lymphoma, basal cell tumour, and prostate cancer.

Autoimmunity occurs when tumour antigens trigger an immune response from the host which creates antibodies that cross react with a retinal protein. This leads to cell apoptosis/death and retinal degeneration.

References

1. Chien JL, Sioufi K, Surakiatchanukul T, Shields JA, Shields CL. Choroidal nevus: a review of prevalence, features, genetics, risks, and outcomes. Curr Opin Ophthalmol. 2017;28(3):228–37.
2. Kaliki S, Shields CL. Uveal melanoma: relatively rare but deadly cancer. Eye (Lond). 2017;31(2):241–57. Published online 2016 Dec 2.
3. Materin MA, Raducu R, Bianciotto C, Shields CL. Fundus autofluorescence and optical coherence tomography findings in choroidal melanocytic lesions. Middle East Afr J Ophthalmol. 2010;17(3):201–6.
4. Wang TW, Liu HW, Bee YS. Distant metastasis in choroidal melanoma with spontaneous corneal perforation and intratumoral calcification: a case report. World J Clin Cases. 2019;7(23):4044–51. https://doi.org/10.12998/wjcc.v7.i23.4044.
5. Laver NV, McLaughlin ME, Duker JS. Ocular melanoma. Arch Pathol Lab Med. 2010;134(12):1778–84.
6. Shields JA, Shields CL. Vascular tumours and malformations of the uvea. In: Atlas of intraocular tumours. Philadelphia: Lippincott, Williams & Wilkins; 2008. p. 230–51.

7. Mashayekhi A, Shields CL. Circumscribed choroidal hemangioma. Curr Opin Ophthalmol. 2003;14:142–9.
8. American Cancer Society. Chapter 85. Neoplasms of the Eye. In: Cancer medicine. Hamilton, Ontario: BC Decker Inc.; 2003. ISBN 978-1-55009-213-4.
9. Ryan SJ.; Schachat AP, Wilkinson CP, Hinton DR, Sadda SVR, Wiedemann P. Retina. Elsevier Health Sciences; 2012. p. 2105. ISBN 978-1455737802.
10. Von Hippel-Lindau disease I Genetic and Rare Diseases Information Centre (GARD)—an NCATS Program. rarediseases.info.nih.gov.
11. Sawyer RA, Selhorst JB, Zimmerman LE, Hoyt WF. Blindness caused by photoreceptor degeneration as a remote effect of cancer. Am J Ophthalmol. 1976;81:606–13.
12. Keltner JL, Roth AM, Chang S. Photoreceptor degeneration—a possible autoimmune disease. Arch Ophthalmol. 1983;101:564–9.

Chapter 10
Retinal Imaging

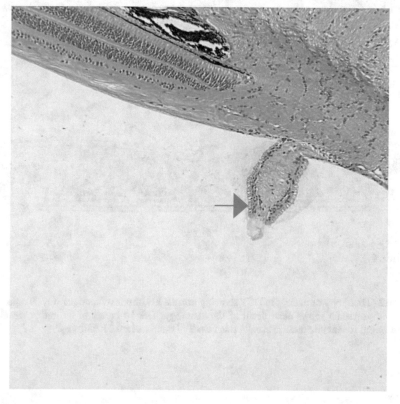

Fig. 10.1 Bergmeister's papilla, arising from the optic disc. Histological section, haematoxylin and eosin stain. Bergmeister's papilla arises from the centre of the optic disc, consists of a small tuft of fibrous tissue (blue arrow) and represents a remnant of the foetal hyaloid artery

© Springer Nature Switzerland AG 2020
M. J. Gouder, *The Retina*, https://doi.org/10.1007/978-3-030-48591-7_10

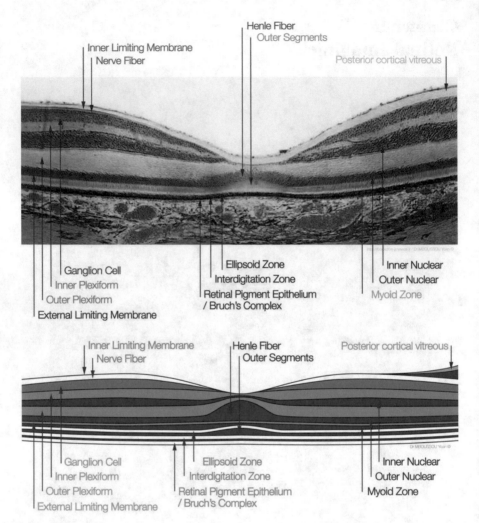

Fig. 10.2 Histology of macula in OCT showing normal healthy fovea and parafoveal area. Illustration in greyscale shows clear detail of the histology. The 10 layers of the retina are clearly seen. Central foveal thickness is usually less than 200 microns in the healthy eye

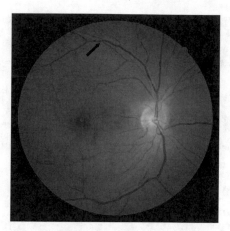

Fig. 10.3 A colour fundus photo of mild hypertensive retinopathy in the right eye showing mild AV nipping denoted by the arrow

Note the prominent focal and generalised arteriolar narrowing. Arrow pointing towards arteriovenous nipping showing venous constriction and banking (see Figs. 10.1, 10.2, 10.3, 10.4, 10.5, 10.6, 10.7, 10.8, 10.9).

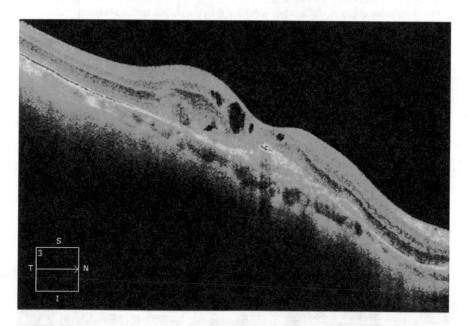

Fig. 10.4 OCT of macula showing disruption of the RPE, a leaking subretinal neovascular membrane with cystic fluid accumulation in the fovea (black arrow) disrupting the local architecture. The patient is a 77 year old female who received multiple intravitreal doses of the anti-VEGF bevacizumab followed by 3 intravitreal doses of aflibercept. Her current BCVA is 6/18 in this eye

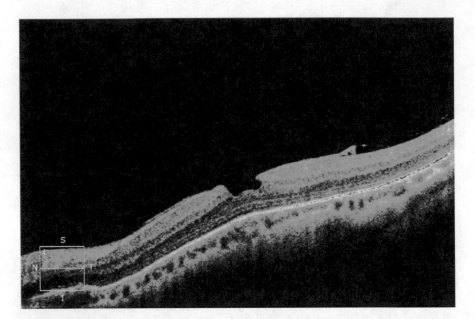

Fig. 10.5 OCT of macula showing a prominent lamellar hole in a 54 year old patient. This is an early degenerative lamellar hole because the foveal edges are not elevated. Note a peculiar non-tractional epimacular tissue which is less reflective than the classic epimacular membrane

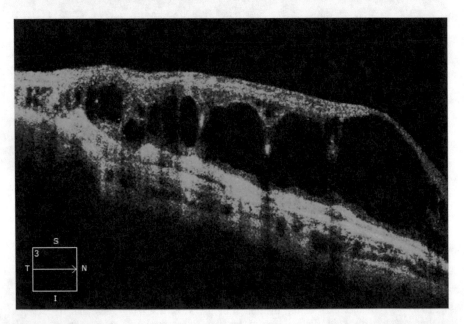

Fig. 10.6 OCT of macula in advanced wet ARMD in a 93 year old woman who received multiple doses of intravitreal bevacizumab. Here we can see complete disruption of the foveal architecture and intraretinal fluid with confluent cystic areas giving the overall thickness of more than 700microns. The visual prognosis is very poor and here the patient is only achieving a BCVA of 6/36. There is also generalised attenuation of the RPE associated with subRPE scarring from long-standing disease

Fig. 10.7 This is an IVFA of the right eye in a patient with central serous retinopathy (CSR). This photo is showing fluorescein leaking from a "hot spot" and pooling in the subretinal space (between RPE and neurosensory retina). This is the classic "smokestack" appearance of CSR

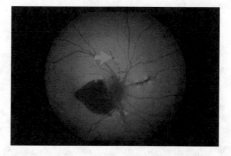

Fig. 10.8 This image showing a fundus autofluorescence (FAF) image showing angioid streaks (blue arrow) radiating out of the optic disc associated with a haemorrhagic leak (red arrow) straddling between the optic disc and the macula. The patient presented with sudden loss of vision in one eye due to this active leak

Fig. 10.9 This is showing a narrow-field image of the same fundus in colour

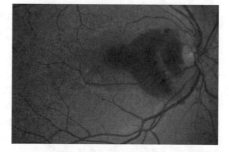

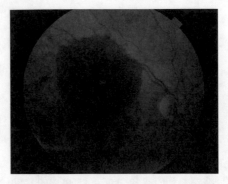

Fig. 10.10   Colour fundus photo of the right eye showing a combination of epiretinal haemorrhage (subhyaloid) inferiorly and the lighter subretinal bleed superiorly. In the latter, one can see prominent vessels still visible because the blood is under the retina. This is caused by an active leak from a SRNVM. The visual prognosis is poor

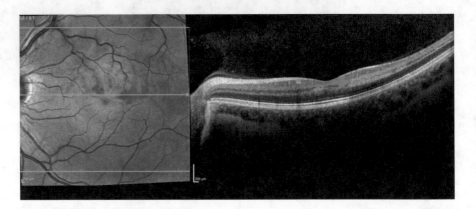

Fig. 10.11   Red-free image (on the left) shows parafoveal hyperreflective specks. Spectral domain OCT analysis (on the right) of the same fundus pathology revealing paracentral acute middle maculopathy (PAMM)

PAMM is a recently recognised entity, as a variant of acute macular neuroretinopathy (AMN), manifesting as hyperreflective band-like lesion (blue arrow) at inner nuclear layer (INL) and outer-plexiform layer (OPL) on spectral domain optical coherence tomography. PAMM is caused by a vascular pathology resulting from ischaemia of deep retinal layers.

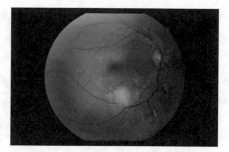

Fig. 10.12 Colour fundus photo of the right eye showing a prominent astrocytoma (blue arrow) in a patient with tuberose sclerosis. A retinal astrocytoma is a rare benign glioma that typically occurs in childhood and adolescence. These are usually asymptomatic unless associated with the macula

Retinal astrocytomas typically appear white in colour, opaque, or translucent, with varying degrees of thickness. Tumours are typically comprised of large, fibrous astrocytes containing small, oval nuclei. Larger tumours may develop areas of calcification. Retinal astrocytomas may be unilateral or bilateral. Patients can sometimes present with an astrocytoma as a manifestation of tuberous sclerosis, which is more commonly seen with bilateral astrocytomas. Retinal astrocytomas rarely become malignant, and treatment is usually observation. Tumours that continue to grow or cause symptoms may require surgical intervention.

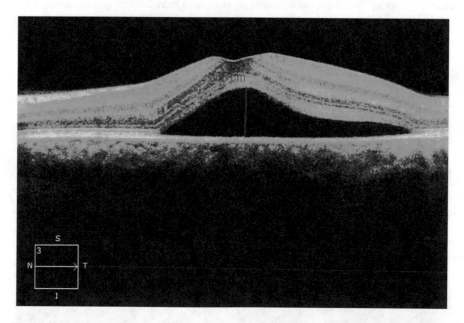

Fig. 10.13 OCT analysis of a macula with a huge central serous retinopathy (CSR). Central serous retinopathy (CSR) is a disease in which a serous detachment of the neurosensory retina occurs over an area of leakage from the choriocapillaris through the retinal pigment epithelium (RPE). It is a self-limited macular disease marked by distortion, blurry vision, and metamorphopsia. In this case the height of the fluid "dome" is measured at 355 microns

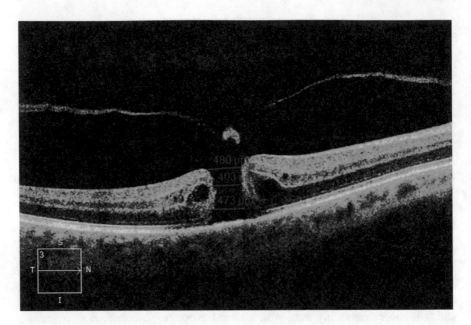

Fig. 10.14 This is an OCT scan of a 55 year old gentleman presenting in the clinic with a full thickness macular hole (FTMH) measuring 480 microns (macular hole inner opening). Base diameter was at around 473 microns. Macular hole inner opening, base diameter and macular hole index are prognostic indicators and determine the anatomical success rate of hole closure after surgery. These indices form the basis for the new international OCT-based classification system for macular holes. The patient underwent a 25G pars plana vitrectomy with ILM peel and C3F8 gas (14%) leading to complete closure of the hole but with a somewhat flattened foveal contour. From 6/60 BCVA the patient achieved 6/9 BCVA. Please see Fig. 10.15 for the post-op OCT image

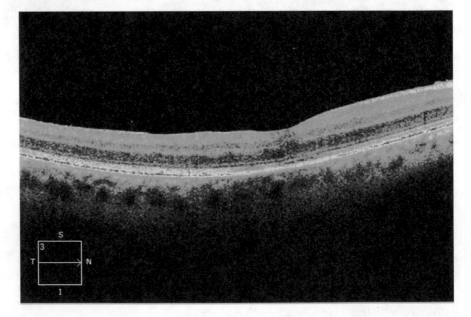

Fig. 10.15 This is the post-operative OCT analysis of the above mentioned patient in Fig. 10.14. One can notice full closure of the FTMH but with a somewhat flat foveal contour

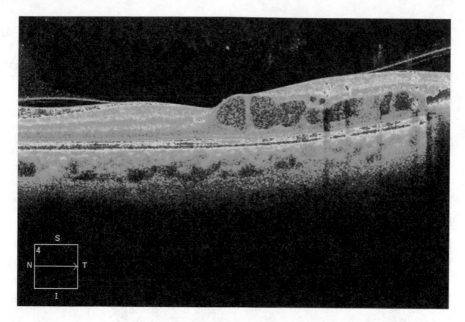

Fig. 10.16 This is an OCT analysis from a female patient with long-standing diabetes associated with metabolic syndrome. The presenting BCVA from this eye was 6/36. The posterior hyaloid face is still attached to the macula but there is asymmetric cystic change in the fovea disrupting the normal formal architecture and contour. This is diabetic macular oedema. The patient was subsequently treated with anti-VEGF therapy improving her BCVA to 6/12+

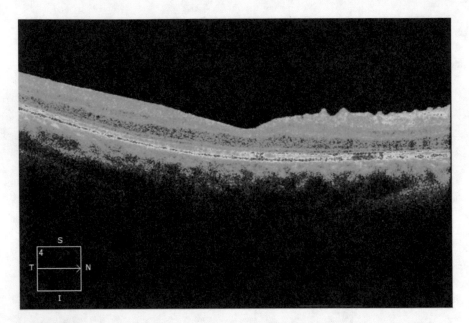

Fig. 10.17 This is an OCT analysis from a 40 year old female patient with long-standing type 1 diabetes. This patient initially presented with proliferative diabetic retinopathy, tractional retinal detachment, profuse fibrovascular fronds and dense vitreous haemorrhage. Her presenting BCVA was 6/60. She underwent a 25G pars plana vitrectomy with membrane peel, endolaser and silicone oil insertion followed by removal of silicone oil and phacoemulsification 6 months later. This OCT shows the post operative result. There is some asymmetrical macular distortion and overall thinning of the retina from the chronic ischaemia. Her final BCVA was 6/12

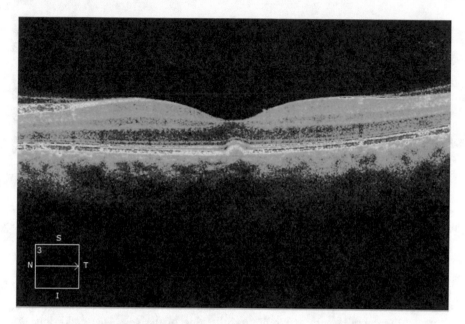

Fig. 10.18 This is an OCT analysis from a 50 year old male asymptomatic patient who was referred by the optometrist because of a small foveal spot detected on routine examination. Clinical examination showed features of a very small pigment epithelial detachment (PED)

The base of a PED is Bruch's membrane and the 'roof' is made up of the RPE. This type is non-vascularised and can be associated with underlying drusen. The OCT is showing this small PED (red arrow). The patient will be monitored with 6 monthly OCT testing.

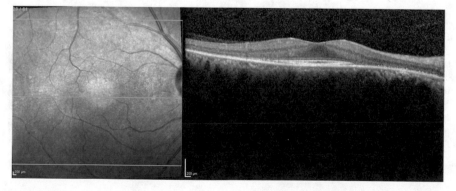

Fig. 10.19 Bull's eye maculopathy caused by hydroxychloroquine (HCQ). The OCT is showing temporal parafoveal thinning and loss of outer segment structural lines

Fig. 10.20 Composite
colour fundus photograph of
a dragged macula in a patient
with familial exudative
vitreoretinopathy (FEVR)

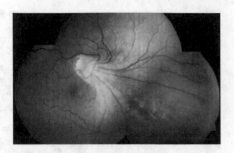

Signs of FEVR;

- Avascular peripheral retina—This can be appreciated on careful fundus examination, however in subtle cases or asymptomatic family members fluorescein
  angiography can be invaluable in uncovering this finding. Classically, the temporal quadrant is most often involved with a v-shaped demarcation. However,
  this a vascularity can extend 360 degrees. In addition, the demarcation is
  described as a "brush-border".
- Dragged retinal vessels and macula—Retinal arteries and veins can be dragged,
  usually temporally with apparent straightening of the vessels. In addition, the
  macula can be dragged temporally.
- Retinal (falciform) folds—Radial retinal folds were seen in 28% of eyes in one
  study. Folds most often are seen in the temporal location, but they can be seen
  in any location.
- Neovascularization—Due to the avascular retina, retinal ischaemia induces
  neovascularization.
- Subretinal exudates—Variable amounts of subretinal exudation can be seen.
  Massive exudation can be seen that can mimic Coat's disease.
- Retinal detachments—Tractional and rhegmatogenous retinal detachments can
  be seen.
- Persistent fetal vasculature.

Fig. 10.21 Colour fundus
photo of the right eye
showing a prominent
choroidal melanoma
involving the inferotemporal
quadrant up to the macula.
Note presence of orange
pigment and some subretinal
fluid

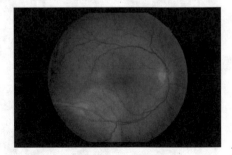

Fig. 10.22 Colour fundus
photo of the right eye
showing a flat choroidal
naevus and associated with
drusen

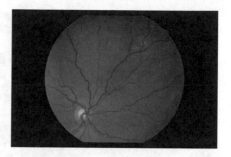

Choroidal nevi tend to have clearly defined margins and to be flat or slightly elevated, and they remain stable in size. Over time, choroidal naevi display features such as overlying drusen as well as retinal pigment epithelial atrophy, hyperplasia or fibrous metaplasia.

In contrast, choroidal melanomas are more likely to show signs of activity such as relatively indiscrete margins, irregular or oblong configuration, overlying subretinal fluid and orange pigment, and abruptly elevated edges.

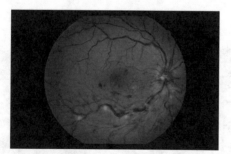

Fig. 10.23 Colour fundus photo of the right eye showing an inferior hemiretinal vein obstruction with macular oedema. This is a 50 year old man with past history of hypertension presenting with 6/60 vision and a superior field defect

Inferiorly one can notice;

- dilated tortuous retinal venules
- retinal oedema associated with ischaemia
- cotton wool spots
- flame-shaped haemorrhages (in NFL)
- microaneurysms.

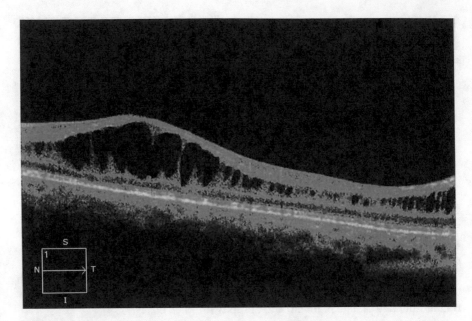

Fig. 10.24 OCT analysis of an 11 year old boy suffering from Juvenile X-linked retinoschisis with a BCVA of 6/36

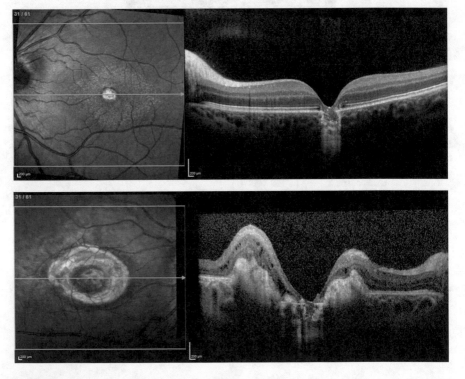

Fig. 10.25 OCT analysis showing North Carolina Dystrophy. Upper image shows Grade 2-3 (yellow drusen-like lesions with larger confluent lesions) whilst the lower image is showing grade 3 pathology (macular colobomatous lesion)

X-linked retinoschisis or juvenile retinoschisis (XLJR) is an inherited disorder affecting only males. It is caused by mutations in the retinoschisin gene (*RS-1*). There is considerable variability in the onset and severity of the disease.

The clinical hallmarks are cystic retinal changes in the macula (stellate maculopathy) and peripheral retinal elevations as the result of retinoschisis.

Vitreous veils over the peripheral schisis, vitreous hemorrhage, and retinal detachment also can occur.

Features of this very rare disease include;

- autosomal dominant
- variable macular phenotype even in the same family
- macular coloboma in 1/3 of patients
- well-demarcated atrophy of the RPE and choriocapillaris
- CNV can complicate the disease.

References

1. Figure 10.1 https://commons.wikimedia.org/wiki/File:Bergmeisters_papilla_x_6.jpg. Licensing: Public Domain Imaging.
2. Figure 10.2 https://commons.wikimedia.org/wiki/File:Macula_Histology_OCT.jpg. Licensing: Public Domain Imaging. Author: Yoan Mboussou.
3. Figure 10.3 https://upload.wikimedia.org/wikipedia/commons/f/ff/Hypertensiveretinopathy. jpg. Frank Wood.
4. Figure 10.4 Obtained from Saint James Eye Hospital OCT library courtesy of MJ Gouder (author).
5. Figure 10.5 Obtained from Saint James Eye Hospital OCT library courtesy of MJ Gouder (author).
6. Figure 10.6 Obtained from Saint James Eye Hospital OCT library courtesy of MJ Gouder (author).
7. Figure 10.7 courtesy of Dr. Alastair Bezzina MD, ChM, FEBO, FICO, MRCSEd(Ophth), Resident Specialist, Mater Dei Hospital, Malta.
8. Figure 10.8 courtesy of Dr. Alastair Bezzina MD, ChM, FEBO, FICO, MRCSEd(Ophth), Resident Specialist, Mater Dei Hospital, Malta.
9. Figure 10.9 courtesy of Dr. Alastair Bezzina MD, ChM, FEBO, FICO, MRCSEd(Ophth), Resident Specialist, Mater Dei Hospital, Malta.
10. Figure 10.10 courtesy of Dr. Alastair Bezzina MD, ChM, FEBO, FICO, MRCSEd(Ophth), Resident Specialist, Mater Dei Hospital, Malta.
11. Figure 10.11 courtesy of Dr. Alastair Bezzina MD, ChM, FEBO, FICO, MRCSEd(Ophth), Resident Specialist, Mater Dei Hospital, Malta.
12. Figure 10.12 courtesy of Dr. Alastair Bezzina MD, ChM, FEBO, FICO, MRCSEd(Ophth), Resident Specialist, Mater Dei Hospital, Malta. Tasman W and Jaeger EA. Atlas of Clinical Ophthalmology. Chapter 7: Retinal Tumours. Ed. 2001: 274–5.
13. Figure 10.13 Obtained from Saint James Eye Hospital OCT library courtesy of MJ Gouder (author).
14. Figure 10.14 Obtained from Saint James Eye Hospital OCT library courtesy of MJ Gouder (author).

15. Figure 10.15 Obtained from Saint James Eye Hospital OCT library courtesy of MJ Gouder (author).
16. Figure 10.16 Obtained from Saint James Eye Hospital OCT library courtesy of MJ Gouder (author).
17. Figure 10.17 Obtained from Saint James Eye Hospital OCT library courtesy of MJ Gouder (author).
18. Figure 10.18 Obtained from Saint James Eye Hospital OCT library courtesy of MJ Gouder (author).
19. Figure 10.19 courtesy of Dr. Alastair Bezzina MD, ChM, FEBO, FICO, MRCSEd(Ophth), Resident Specialist, Mater Dei Hospital, Malta.
20. Figure 10.20 courtesy of Dr. James Vassallo MD, MRCSEd, FICO, FEBO, MRCSEd(Ophth) and Dr. Suzanne Pirotta MD, MRCOphth, FEBO, Resident Specialists, Mater Dei Hospital, Malta. https://eyewiki.aao.org/Familial_Exudative_Vitreoretinopathy_(FEVR).
21. Figure 10.21 Obtained from Mater Dei Hospital, Malta, Fundus Camera library courtesy of MJ Gouder (author). OPHTHALMIC PEARLS from www.aao.org. Distinguishing a Choroidal Nevus From a Choroidal Melanoma, Written By: Albert Cheung, Ingrid U. Scott, MD, MPH, Timothy G. Murray, MD, and Carol L. Shields, MD, Edited by Ingrid U. Scott, MD, MPH, and Sharon Fekrat, MD.
22. Figure 10.22 Obtained from Mater Dei Hospital, Malta, Fundus Camera library courtesy of MJ Gouder (author). OPHTHALMIC PEARLS from www.aao.org. Distinguishing a Choroidal Nevus From a Choroidal Melanoma, Written By: Albert Cheung, Ingrid U. Scott, MD, MPH, Timothy G. Murray, MD, and Carol L. Shields, MD, Edited by Ingrid U. Scott, MD, MPH, and Sharon Fekrat, MD.
23. Figure 10.23 Obtained from Mater Dei Hospital, Malta, Fundus Camera library courtesy of MJ Gouder (author).
24. Figure 10.24 Obtained from Saint James Eye Hospital OCT library courtesy of MJ Gouder (author).
25. Figure 10.25 courtesy of Dr. Alastair Bezzina MD, ChM, FEBO, FICO, MRCSEd(Ophth), Resident Specialist, Mater Dei Hospital, Malta. Macular Dystrophy, Retinal, 1, North Carolina Type; MCDR1. Online Mendelian Inheritance in Man (OMIM). August 11, 2016.

Index

© Springer Nature Switzerland AG 2020
M. J. Gouder, *The Retina*, https://doi.org/10.1007/978-3-030-48591-7

Printed in the United States
by Baker & Taylor Publisher Services